Chronic Disease Diet: The Complete Guide to Losing Weight, Improving Sleep, and Fighting Chronic Inflammation

David Friedman, PharmD

TABLE OF CONTENTS

<u>Lose Weight And Prevent Heart Disease, Stroke, Cancer, And Type 2 Diabetes With These Doctor-Approved Methods</u>

What are you afraid of?

Dying in a road accident? Being killed by a terrorist? Being eaten by a shark?

But did you know that you're much, much more risk to die of stroke or a heart attack?

Chronic illnesses like heart disease, obesity, and diabetes kill more people worldwide than wars and accidents do. It's true that doctors are getting better and better at doing complex surgeries, healing terrible injuries, and helping chronically ill people lead longer, better lives. However, they can't do as much when it comes to **preventing** disease.

Very often, your lifestyle is your best medicine.

Even small changes can have benefit effects. If you sleep more than 6 hours a night, you can reduce your risk of heart disease by 20% just **by adopting better sleep strategies**. A **single change to your**

diet will reduce your risk of diabetes-related complications by 44% (even if you've already been diagnosed with the disease).

As you see, simple lifestyle hacks can literally prevent disability and early death.

In this book, pharmacist David Friedman will reveal the newest medical advice on preventing and managing chronic disease with four natural tools: diet, sleep, stress management, and controlling inflammation. His recommendations are highly practical and actionable so that you can start boosting your health and preventing terrible diseases right away.

Here's what you'll learn:

- **The sad TRUTH about popular weight loss diets – and how to lose weight the right way**

- Scientifically proven workouts to maximize weight loss and boost your heart health

- **How smart sleep strategies reduce your risk of cancer, diabetes, and autoimmune diseases**

- Natural methods to control inflammation, the mother of all disease

- **How to minimize the symptoms of chronic disease if you've already been diagnosed**

This book is all about serious and scientifically correct medical advice. It's not trying to sell you anything – instead, it seeks to empower you to make healthy lifestyle choices.

Reclaim control of your health NOW, before it's too late.

YOU CAN BE YOUR OWN MEDICINE

Who doesn't want to enjoy a pleasant life, as long as possible and in good health? Cycling again at 100 with your grandkids? This is possible if only you make this choice first. For example, we do not suspect how much excess weight can sneak up on us for chronic diseases while eating away at our life expectancy. And yet, we are in the front seat of a global explosion of these diseases. They have a major impact on our quality of life and lead to physical and moral suffering with serious consequences. They also lead to premature deaths and impact the economic strength of families. These are particularly cardiovascular diseases, cancer, respiratory diseases and type 2 diabetes. In the United States [1], the number of people with chronic diseases increased in 2005 from 133 million (46.2% of the population) to 149 million (47.3% of the population). Projections for 2030 are estimated at 171 million (49.2% of the population). In Europe, despite the overall increase in life expectancy observed around 2017 [2], the number of cancer cases per year is estimated at 3.91 million in 2018 [3], compared to an estimated 3.2 million in 2008 [4].

In the performance of my duties, the observation of this increase in chronic pathologies seemed obvious to me. As a clinical pharmacist, I have collaborated with various interveners in the hospital world, including doctors of all specialties (general practitioners, cardiologists, pulmonologists, nephrologists, diabetologists, oncologists, etc.) as well as with the administrative and economic services of the institution.

My daily routine with my fellow doctors is to provide them with pharmaceutical advice in connection with increasingly complex clinical cases. Over the years, patients become polypathological and therefore require heavy care. Each medication prescribed at the right time, at the right dose, responded to a specific pathology. In hospitals, where patients are in critical situations, the choice of medication must be carefully considered. Patients sometimes have kidney failure, or are already on other medications that can complicate their situation. Over the years, I have observed that the number of meds patients take on a daily basis is increasing. As a result, the number of meds per prescription for the management of these chronic diseases is reaching alarming levels. A survey conducted in France in 2017 revealed that patients over 65 years of age have an average of 14 different meds on their prescriptions. They are, therefore, exposed to a medication deluge with the risk of serious adverse reactions that can lead to repeated hospitalizations. During hospitalization, a patient with several illnesses (type 2 diabetes, hypertension, heart failure, anxiety, etc.) is often examined by several specialist doctors, which keeps them totally dependent on many meds and care. In the United States, the polymedication is so acute that it is estimated that for every 1000 people admitted to the emergency room, 4 people are admitted, just because of the adverse effects of meds (mainly anticoagulants, insulin, painkillers and antibiotics)[5]. In 2015, the opiate epidemic killed 52,000 people in the USA[6], surpassing the fatal accidents caused by cars. In 2017, in the State of Maryland, Governor Larry Hogan had to declare a state of emergency to counter the phenomenon[7]. Even the President of the US Federal Reserve has expressed concern about the negative impact of the phenomenon on the entire US economy[8].

Despite medical developments, things do not seem to be moving in the brighter direction. Despite the therapeutic arsenal, the care, the increasingly sophisticated diagnostic tools, the causes of most pathologies are not treated in depth. Discomfort remains an issue. In-depth treatment certainly requires a great deal of involvement with the patient. It seems obvious that to cure the ills suffered by human beings, it is necessary to priorily investigate their living conditions. It is obvious that prevention is excessively lacking and that once the disease has been declared, medicine does not yet have the answer to all situations. For example, depression can no longer be bundled up as a single theory that is a deficit or low production of serotonin in the brain. If this were the case, all meds or therapies intended to increase this neurotransmitter in the brain would have been very successful in the management of depression.

Another example is the understanding of Alzheimer's disease, a disease characterized by memory disorders, where a lot remains to be discovered. For decades, the theory of a neurotransmitter deficiency, acetylcholine, was the " core " of the management of Alzheimer patients. Patients were treated with "acetylcholinesterase inhibitors" either in tablet form or as devices to be glued to the skin. These drugs are intended to increase the production of acetylcholine in the brain. It has to be said that these long-term drugs are practically useless, especially when the disease is severe and these drugs are more likely to cause serious or even fatal adverse reactions[9]. Let us be clear, it is by no means a question of rejecting the progress of medicine in its entirety, but of becoming aware that it is possible, by means of simple rules, to avoid complicated situations.

In my daily practice, I have seen how the introduction of new antivirals against hepatitis C has cured patients who were previously treated with interferons, with no hope for a real cure, and who were also experiencing extremely distressing side effects. The availability of these antivirals is a major therapeutic breakthrough. In my opinion, the patients' healing is almost spectacular! Another example is the management of children with a rare deficiency of a protein that enables blood clotting, factor 5. These cases are different from the classic hemophilia we often hear about. These children were subject to blood spills in the knee joints, and received plasma transfusions. They were faced with serious allergic problems. It was from the pharmaceutical industry that a new healthy plasma arrived that was able to solve these allergy problems and save the lives of these children. And that's just to name a few...

The management of patients can sometimes be extremely time-consuming and complex. It often happens that diseases recur, and patients find themselves in a path of struggle that exhausts them. Except for acute pathologies, which for the most part require care of about ten days to be cured, chronic pathologies generally last more than 6 months, and require complex care. In chronic diseases, the doctor seeks to slow the progression of the disease by controlling it. Sometimes surgery or radiotherapy techniques come in handy. It is not uncommon for treatments to get heavier over time. For persistent chest pain, a medically managed patient may find himself or herself with five medications to ingest daily over time. There is no guarantee that they can withstand these treatments, not to mention the impact they could have on their daily life. If we take chemotherapy, for example, great progress has been made over the past few years. With the advent of monoclonal antibodies, patient management is becoming more targeted and adverse events are less severe. Nevertheless, these treatments still have limitations, their effectiveness decreases over time and, above all, they only work on a limited number of patients. Sometimes, adverse reactions may appear up to 5 months after stopping treatment. These situations force doctors to return to the old anti-cancer molecules that act directly on DNA and have extremely serious adverse effects on patients. Nausea, vomiting, total weakening of the immune system and infections that eventually lead to death. As a clinical pharmacist accompanying oncologists to validate the appropriateness of prescribed treatments, these times when treatments no longer work are a particularly difficult experience.

It is clear that we stand a better chance of promoting a preventive health policy. Similarly, once a disease is diagnosed, changing our way of life can radically change the course of the disease. For type 2 diabetes, for example, once diagnosed, a person who reduces daily caloric intake by 300 calories or more reduces complications of the disease and mortality by 44%[10]. To get the best results, especially for chronic diseases, it is essential to clearly identify the most important risk factors that cause these diseases. Caring for a patient suffering from Crohn's disease requires knowledge of his or her lifestyle, in short, everything that characterizes the individual. If the factors triggering the attacks of the disease are not identified, the patient may recur repeatedly and find themselves in a therapeutic escalation or worse in a dead end where no medication would work. For the patient, we would be compelled to move towards heavy and costly interventions. In Crohn's disease, it is estimated that more than 90% of patients will require an intervention and that for more than 50%, a second intervention, with heavy surgical procedures, is required[11].

Another example is the case of high blood pressure, one of the most common diseases in the world. It is estimated that more than one billion adults will be affected by 2025[12]. These cardiovascular consequences degrade the quality of life of patients[13] and lead to 8 million deaths per year worldwide despite the available therapeutic measures[14]. And yet, there are simple preventive strategies that can slow down, or even prevent, the onset of this disease. Unfortunately, it is only when things get complicated that we become aware of preventive solutions. If we take the case of prostate cancer, which is widespread in Europe and the United States, few men know that consuming mushrooms from the age of 50, and at least 3 times a week, is a simple way to reduce the risk of this cancer[15]. As illustrated with these examples, we have the opportunity to take control of our health to avoid these complex situations. All you have to do is act early enough. Modern life puts us in various risk situations that constantly threaten our well-being.

Nevertheless, we are now fortunate to have access to quality information on a permanent basis. In writing this book, I have set myself the primary objective of clarifying those who are seeking the essentials of information, to live a modern life, while preserving their health through simple principles.

HOW TO READ AND UNDERSTAND THE APPROACH OF THIS BOOK?

This book is organized around 4 main themes, which I consider to be the important factors to which we must pay attention every day and from now on when we read this book. These points are directly related to our quality of life. The threat that looms on each point can have one or more consequences on our lives. The effect can be immediate or insidious. In the long term, they are extremely harmful to our health, our economic strength, and well-being in general.

These 4 essential points are WEIGHT, STRESS, SLEEP, and INFLAMMATION. My entire approach is based on a detailed bibliography, sometimes with real cases. At each point, I detail the failures caused on our body and how to prevent them on a daily and long-term basis.

At the end of the book, a concise summary of the actions to be taken to minimize these failures is described. The form is always based on rules from scientific journals. The daily application of these rules must yield the expected results. It is a question of adopting a global approach, not separate measures. Sleep duration, for example, is a determining factor for health, and this applies to everyone. You can follow all possible diets, for good heart health or to avoid Alzheimer's disease, if you sleep less than 6 hours a night, you increase your risk of heart attack by 20% compared to the person who sleeps between 7 and 8 hours a night, and who eats normally without particularly paying attention t their diet. By depriving yourself of sleep, despite a diet based on the healthiest products, you increase the risk of having bad cholesterol[16]. The book's approach is based on small measures to be implemented on a daily basis. It is not a question of providing methods to lose 15 kg in 60 days but of providing solutions that are almost unconscious and that can be gradually integrated into everyday life. As everyone knows, sudden changes can hardly be sustained in the long term. They are sometimes dangerous to our health. Radical, brutal solutions, promising mountains and wonders in record time, motivate enormously but are difficult to obtain, because they require immense efforts. It is easier to set your goals in several steps, without delay, at the risk of starting to secrete cortisol. For example, when you have to do 5 physical exercise sessions of 10 minutes per week, start with 2 sessions per week, then 3 per week, then 5 per week. As for the diet, it is not a question of no longer enjoying yourself by refusing to consume festive dishes offered during an evening with friends, for example. It is the daily diet that is the objective to be improved. And the results will be even better with regular physical exercise.

Whether you are in Washington, London or Sydney... you can put into practice the solutions proposed in this book, for your physical and mental health.

WEIGHT

Weight is one of the cardinal points impacting our health. It is a major issue when it comes to health control. Excess weight is a risk factor in the occurrence of many diseases. Globally, the number of overweight adults is estimated at 1.9 billion, 650 million of whom are obese[17].

The difference between obesity and overweight is simple. It is derived from the calculation of the BMI (Body Mass Index). Many websites provide a simple automated calculator to calculate BMI. It is just a matter of dividing the weight in kilograms by the square of the height. Depending on the figure obtained, any individual can reliably know whether they are of normal weight (if BMI between 18 and 25) or overweight (between 25 and 30) or obese >30.

Did you know? Although the BMI is considered outdated, it is still used in most published studies. Currently, the best health index is considered to be the waist/hip ratio, which takes into account the distribution of fat over the body. Significant abdominal fat is a deleterious factor for cardiovascular health, and is taken into account by this new indicator. This ratio measures waist and hip circumference, with women not exceeding 0.7 and men not exceeding 0.9. If values are exceeded, diet and exercise should be controlled.

Apart from the health impact and consequences of overweight, the economic cost of obesity is very high. These expenses are directly correlated to the management of all the resulting pathologies. In the United States alone, it is estimated that 215 billion dollars are spent annually on obesity care[18]. But where the subject is becoming alarming, is that the percentage of obese people will continue to increase by 2030.

Being overweight reduces our life expectancy by 4 years

Many people are unaware of this, but being overweight lowers our life expectancy. A relationship is established between obesity and premature death. A study involving more than 3 million people shows that when BMI is either too low or too high, life expectancy drops by 4 years![19] And one of the conclusions of this study is that when you have a BMI between 22 and 25, life expectancy remains unchanged compared to official estimates. Although BMI has some weaknesses as a physiological indicator, the objective of any individual should be to maintain their BMI within this ideal range of 22-25.

Being overweight increases the risk of cardiovascular disease and type 2 diabetes.

A BMI > 30 increases the risk of cardiovascular diseases such as myocardial infarction, stroke, heart failure and even sudden death[20]. The aggravating factor is the presence of visceral obesity, which is located in the abdomen. In this case, it is an accumulation of fatty tissues, which acts as an organ secreting aggravating factors of cardiovascular diseases. The factors secreted by this abdominal tissue disrupt the coagulability of the blood and potentiate myocardial infarction[21].

Thus, a high BMI coupled with an abdominal circumference (>80 cm for women and 102 cm for men)[22] is a high cardiovascular risk situation. Anyone who has an abdominal circumference value exceeding the indicated figure should consider calculating their waist/hip ratio. The result will allow you to review your daily diet and implement measures to be more active. Similarly, obesity is a very high risk factor for type 2 diabetes. It has been clearly demonstrated in obese women over 100 kg that a BMI > 35 doubles the risk of type 2 diabetes and that a simple weight loss of 5 kg certainly reduces this risk by half[23].

More recently, the link between obesity and disease has been validated in adults for the majority of chronic diseases[24].

Did you know? Type 2 diabetes is a chronic disease, characterized by a lack or deficiency of insulin. It is characterized by the body's resistance to the effects of insulin. Insulin is a hormone produced by the pancreas that allows glucose to enter the blood, adipose tissue, liver, and muscles. When insulin cannot perform its function, glucose accumulates in the blood: this is called hyperglycemia. In the medium to long term, this hyperglycemia can cause complications, especially in the eyes, kidneys, nerves, heart and blood vessels.

Being overweight increases the risk of cancer

There is a very strong relationship between BMI and cancer occurrence. Several types of cancer are involved, and the general public is not sufficiently informed about this link between obesity and cancer. For breast cancer, for example, studies have shown that the risk is increased in obese postmenopausal women[25]. The cause is believed to be high estrogen levels. In premenopausal obese women, the estimated risks are low. What is special about obese postmenopausal women is that the abdominal fat tissue secretes a growth factor called IGF (Insulin-like Growth Factor). IGF is normally secreted by the liver, but in cases of obesity, abdominal fat tissue becomes a production centre, resulting in the proliferation of cancer cells[26]. All these phenomena are self-sustaining by stimulating macrophages that release substances to activate the birth of cancer cells. Excess weight is also involved in digestive cancers. And it is the whole digestive sphere that can be affected, namely the colon, liver, stomach, pancreas, esophagus... In France, the French Association of Surgery is calling for a prevention plan for people at risk, because surgeons have noticed that the risk of developing these digestive cancers is 2 to 5 times higher among obese people.

Other cancers such as endometrial, prostate and other cancers are linked to obesity. It is important that this information is known, because once the cancer disease is declared, the value of weight loss is no longer obvious.

The good news is that weight is a modifiable risk factor. It is possible for everyone to take action to counteract all the harmful effects of overweight and obesity. Diets have failed 80% of the time. This is not a lack of will, but as neurobiologist Traci Mann explains so well, neurological, hormonal and metabolic phenomena automatically develop, to attract us to an even more appetizing and delicious food, when we start a diet. The ideal solution would be to put in place smart, progressive, low-binding and sustainable solutions to bring BMI back into the normal range.

Diet as a key factor and its interaction with the brain

Diet is a very important factor in weight reduction because every day we provide calories to the body for our physiological balance. Controlling food involves very complex processes whose understanding is essential. Without a balanced diet, you can do all the necessary sports activity, your weight loss results will be poor or even zero in the long term! Eating is a pleasant experience that involves processes of rewards, emotions and memory in the brain... Each time a food substance is ingested, the nerve centres receive stimuli that are considered rewards. Overall, these rewards can be translated in two ways: The first is energy balance or homeostasis, the purpose of which is to maintain a balanced caloric energy balance. The main aim is to compensate for calorie expenditure by providing calories. The second, the hedonic reward is much more related to the pleasure derived from taste or smell... The combination of these two systems determines our eating behaviour. Chemical intermediates, one of the most important of which is insulin, govern our relationship to food. Controlling insulin secretion, through diet and physical activity, is the key to controlling our weight. Anything that reduces the amount of insulin secreted by the pancreas is a weight control solution. Some people are able to control their food intake without much effort, and therefore avoid unnecessary and superfluous calories. For others, it is a real obstacle course. No discouragement, the problem is well known and has been the subject of much research, it is quite possible to modify one's eating behavior, in order to reduce one's weight in the long term. These solutions will gradually control your appetite and the effects will be significant in the long term.

What would reduce weight in the long term? Do not set a time limit and do not use much insulin from the pancreas.

There is a set of elements that must be taken into account to answer this question. Losing weight, without upsetting our body, is possible. As already mentioned, failure rates are high and dropouts are high. These failures are due to the fact that each organism has its balance, any intervention faces a cascade of events through hormones to return to the initial state. For example, when we reduce the intake of calories absorbed daily, hormonal mechanisms will initially stimulate appetite to compensate for this sudden caloric disruption. It is therefore necessary to stimulate the body to a new balance, which necessarily requires time. The winning strategy is to put all the necessary conditions in place, so that the efforts required can be used less to solicit compensation mechanisms. What are these mechanisms and how can we reduce their activation?

The first thing is not to set a deadline for losing weight. When you set a time limit such as: "I have to lose 5 kg in 15 days", and start the diet under these conditions, you automatically and unconsciously trigger the secretion of cortisol and betatrophin[27], the stress hormone and the rapid multiplication of insulin-producing cells, which push you to seek food to compensate for this stress. Again, don't set a deadline, just determine how you will gradually make yourself more active.

The second thing is to avoid any stimulation of insulin secretion. Insulin is a hormone secreted by the pancreas, which has the primary role of regulating blood glucose levels. It is a matter of adopting all the solutions so as not to ask your pancreas for insulin secretion. There are two ways to do this: reduce the carbohydrates you ingest, especially fast carbohydrates, and exercise, in short, move as much as possible. If the rapid decrease in carbohydrates is not achieved, there will be an abundance of food, and the insulin released will automatically convert the carbohydrates into fatty acids, which are then stored in the adipocytes and contribute to the increase in weight. Keep in mind that adipocytes are real fat storage stores on the stomach and thighs, where they can increase in volume up to 100 times! Of course, you can significantly reduce carbohydrates (50 gr per day instead of 200 gr), and make the muscles and brain work with a high proportion of lipids (meat or vegetable fats). By doing this, you will lose weight, up to 12 kg on average between 3 and 12 months, but in most cases, you will be tired after 2 years, and if you do not resist, the weight will go up very quickly. For the majority of people who try to eat a high-fat diet after one or two years, weight loss is often between 1 and 3 kg. For an individual weighing 105 kg, this is not much in relation to the time and effort involved[28]. In the long term, these low-carbohydrate diets do not impact weight, and the results are even similar to a normal diet[29][30]. Worse still, for those who can continue for years, the risk of death from cardiovascular disease is high[31]. What diet should be adopted to lose weight in the long term?

Meals rich in fibre for a hunger suppressant and protective effect on the intestinal flora

Very often, patients are rushed to hospital for constipation or obstruction of the intestine. Apart from the drugs and age that can induce these problems, it is the low fruit and vegetable diet that is often the cause. A varied diet rich in vegetables and fruit is essential for transit but also for weight control. This involves reducing the proportion of fast carbohydrates and replacing them with whole or semi-soft foods (wholegrain bread, wholegrain rice, whole or semi-soft pasta for starchy foods). Vegetables and fruit alone provide a significant amount of carbohydrates for the body. They can grow large enough in the stomach to stimulate satiety receptors. It is also important to choose fruits and vegetables that are pleasant to the taste, to ensure the pleasure of eating. When the meal contains enough vegetables, it is not necessary to count the calories contained in the meals. Overall, vegetables and fruit must make up at least 60% of the total meal. Of course, a person who has a diet rich in vegetables and fruit and lacks physical activity will only slightly reduce their weight[32]. Indeed, an observation of 1026 individuals who did not receive specific advice and were just encouraged to consume fruit and vegetables for weeks clearly shows a decrease of 0.54 kg per individual, which is low[33]. Most people have no clear idea of the daily intake of fruits and vegetables they need. The Western diet provides an average of 15 grams of fibre per day, which corresponds to about 100 grams of vegetables and fruit per day. This is extremely low. Fibres also called fibers are plant residues that the body cannot digest because they are not degraded by the enzymes in the human digestive tract. Weight loss can be improved by incorporating higher proportions of vegetables and fruit containing at least 30 g of fibre per day into the diet[34 35]. This corresponds to at least 200 g of green vegetables per day. As you can see, you need to eat even more food to ensure weight loss, but be careful with adequate food. Under these conditions, without stress, anyone can expect a loss of up to 5 kg after 2 years of a high-fibre diet[36]. A daily intake of vitamin B12 (only present in products of animal origin) should not be neglected, as people who avoid any products of animal origin in their diet, such as meat, fish, eggs or cheese, have a 20% increased risk of stroke[37].

It is then legitimate to wonder by what mechanism, the more than 30 grams of fiber can reduce an individual's weight? The interest of fibres is not only in regulating transit. A first explanation can be found in the modification of the intestinal flora, i.e. all the bacteria living in perfect symbiosis in the digestive tract. These billions of bacteria contained in our digestive tract are involved in regulating our weight. A prolonged change in our diet can affect the intestinal flora. Consumption of more than 30 g of daily fibre increases the number of bacteroidetes and actinobacteria in the colon, which are bacteria found mainly in individuals of low weight[38]. Similarly, in children aged 4 to 8 years, it has been clearly demonstrated that eating 2 servings of fruit providing at least 2.5 g of fibre per serving stimulates the growth of bifidobacteria and that after 6 months, there is a reduction in the bad bacteria involved in diarrhoea. All this naturally contributes to the well-being of the child[39]. Similarly, inside vegetables, there may be bacteria that balance the flora: an apple, for example, contains millions of bacteria, whether biological or not, and contrary to what one might think, it is inside the apples, i.e. in the pulp, that there is a large part of the bacteria[40]. Fruits and vegetables provide us with bacteria that help us to have a more varied and protective microbiota.

A second explanation is that fruits and vegetables contain few calories, and can have a volumetric effect that increases satiety. They have the ability to absorb water with their fibres and therefore have a hunger suppressant effect. This effect is complex and involves the upper nerve centres, intestines and hormonal mediators[41]. Dietary fibre, which has a high viscosity, can have this hunger suppressant effect in most individuals[42]. It is therefore necessary to favour fruits and vegetables, rich in fibre, having a very good taste, and arousing a real pleasure in eating. The avocado, for example, consumed on a regular basis can give significant results. It is rich in nutrients and considered moderately high in calories[43]. Half an avocado provides 160 calories and 7gr of fibre. It is consumed raw and thus restores all its nutrients. A study including more than 17,000 individuals consuming half an avocado per day and followed for 7 years, shows that the average weight is 78 kg, with a low BMI (26.7) and a non-excessive abdominal volume (93.2 cm), compared to the non-consumers. Consuming half or a whole avocado per day limits weight gain and obesity[43 44].

When it comes to weight loss, the consumption of certain fruits and vegetables must be limited. These are mainly potatoes, maize and peas, which rather contribute to an increase in weight[45]. Thanks to rigorous monitoring of the daily consumption of fruit and vegetables, the researchers have classified fruit and vegetables in order to significantly reduce weight over the long term. It shows that blueberries, cauliflower, apple, pear, green beans are excellent for weight loss. Broccoli, pepper, avocado and carrot also help you lose weight.

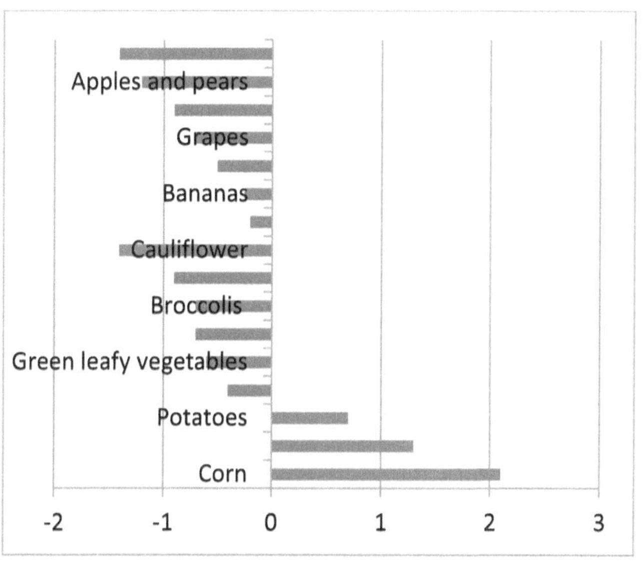

Variation in body weight (Ibs) after daily consumption for 4 years[45]

Drink 2 x 125 ml glasses of water before each meal

Drinking water before each meal is a simple way to quickly reach satiety. Drinking 500 ml of water just before the start of the meal reduces the calories consumed[46]. Weight loss can reach 2 kg after 12 weeks without any stress[47]. The water ingested before meals acts as a satiating effect, simply stimulating the satiety receptors in the stomach wall. It is essential to give up sweetened drinks and gradually develop the habit of drinking 2 glasses of water before meals. From my own experience, even if 500 ml of water before meals seems to me to be a lot to hold on to over time, drinking about 250 ml of water before and 250 ml during meals is a possible objective. The practice becomes routine and, over time, it becomes even strange and tasteless to accompany meals with sweetened drinks. And we see the interest in abandoning these sweetened drinks, when we know that ingesting 100 ml of sweetened drinks per day increases the risk of cancer by 18%[48].

Regular physical activity to keep your metabolism active

Regular physical activity is the key to weight loss. All studies attest to this. To fully understand the situation, a number of simple elements and figures should be retained. Every day, a man needs an average of 2800 calories and a woman 2200 calories. The crux of the problem is that we are becoming more and more sedentary, while absorbing many calories. In the USA, for example, it has been noted over a 20-year period that the proportion of women reporting no physical activity has increased from 19.1% to 51.7%, and for men from 11.4% to 43.5%. Very importantly, during this period, BMI and abdominal circumference increased very significantly[49] Any awakening situation characterized by a very low energy expenditure is harmful to our body. However, the figures are alarming: adults are becoming more and more sedentary, with an average of more than 9 hours of inactivity per day[50][51]. And be careful, just because you're active doesn't mean you're not sedentary. There are "sedentary actives". This is the typical case of the office employee who remains seated all day long.

James Levine, an American endocrinologist, made it clear in 2014 in the Los Angeles Time that "sitting is more dangerous than smoking and kills more than HIV "[52]. Apart from the increase in weight, the damage associated with the decrease in physical activity is considerable and devious. The lack of regular physical activity is related to cardiovascular diseases, type 2 diabetes and cancer[53][54]. A person who works in a sitting position for more than 10 hours a day increases the risk of death by 34%, regardless of age[55]. In terms of life expectancy, sitting less than 3 hours a day is a gain of 2 years of life in addition [56]. We are at a time when, despite the availability of information on the factors that threaten our health, we are adopting an increasingly harmful lifestyle. The modern environment favours a sedentary lifestyle. Some experts argue that from a degree of sedentariness, generally more than 10 hours a day, the damage caused to our body is irreversible, regardless of the measures adopted to limit this damage. Fortunately, studies show that solutions exist. Moderate and regular physical activity reduces mortality. By moving as much as possible, we strengthen our overall health without costing us a cent. In today's world, to enjoy better health in the long term, we need to be physically active on a regular basis and move as much as possible.

Walk, climb stairs and move as much as possible

A few years ago, I was prone to repetitive hemorrhoids. I didn't pay much attention to it because they were healing on their own. Then over time, they came back and caught my attention. I linked them to my coffee consumption. It was only when they persisted longer that I began to look for the cause. Despite well monitored treatments, they came back. That's when I made a link with the number of hours of physical inactivity. Between the car, the desk and in the evenings sitting in an armchair, I practically lived seated. Things then improved when I decided to integrate more walking into my weekend activities. To my great surprise, I noticed a weight loss of 2 kg after one month, walking 3 hours on weekends. I hadn't even changed my eating habits. What was nice was that I felt that walking connected me again to my body. On weekend mornings, there is little car traffic and practically no noise. Equipped with comfortable shoes, I had just downloaded into my smartphone, an application that calculated my number of steps through the alleys and parks. My walking was of moderate intensity, which allowed me to do it for 1 hour and a half a day without a real feeling of exhaustion. At the end of the walk, instead of taking the elevator, I simply took the stairs, which required a more intensive final effort. Morally, I felt better too.

Let us go back to the 1964 Olympic Games. A company, Yamasa Corporation, launches a pedometer called the Manpo-kei, which means "Let's walk 10,000 steps a day". Thus, after the games, the researcher Yoshiro Hatano, measured that 10,000 steps burned 300 calories. While this figure of "10,000 steps per day" has become popular today, additional data provide us with indications of the number of steps that can impact our health. A study shows that around 7500 steps per day, the mortality rate decreases, and that the intensity of walking has little impact on this result[57]. Thanks to my smartphone, I knew that, concretely 7500 steps a day, at a moderate pace, represents about 6 km covered in 1 hour with 400 calories expended.

But what exactly is the deal, when it comes to weight? How many steps do you need each day to lose weight? What amount of weight can we expect to lose by walking for 1 hour a day? The results of a study carried out on a diet for 88 overweight individuals show that 30 or 60 minutes of walking, 5 times a week in combination with a diet, results in a 5.8 kg weight loss in 3 months[58]. Analyses carried out on larger samples show that regular walking, 20 to 60 minutes, 2 to 7 times a week, without taking into account a diet, allows for a weight loss of 1.37 kg from the 8th week[59 60]. As we can see, the results are even more interesting in the context of a diet.

Beyond the impact on weight, the effect is very positive on cardiovascular and respiratory diseases: blood pressure, the volume of oxygen consumed, the circumference of the abdomen is gradually improved by regular and prolonged walking[60]. Unfortunately, modern life condemns us to a level of sedentary life exceeding 9 hours a day. With a simple smartphone app for quantifying our number of steps, you can integrate regular walking into your daily routine, and get an idea of how many calories you can burn just by walking. To do this, you can take advantage of certain situations to reduce your level of sedentary life: taking the stairs gives you even more interesting results. This is proven, and highly recommended by researchers. Climbing stairs is an estimated caloric loss of 14 calories per minute[61]. Take advantage of any situation that you get, to use the stairs at least three times a day. There are no limits... on the street, at work, at the station, at home, when getting out of the subway, take the stairs. Imagine the cumulative effect after 3 months, for a person who takes the stairs every day to get out of the subway, compared to a person who does not take them. The researchers are positive: everyone can improve their physical condition by applying this simple trick. Sedentary adults improved their cardiac and respiratory conditions in a record 6 weeks, using the stairs regularly[62]. The explanation lies in the fact that taking the stairs forces us to do short, intense exercises that very quickly improve our cardiorespiratory functions.

Another possibility is to simply use your car less, if that's possible. The improvement in physical fitness can be dramatic. Leaving your car would cancel out the harmful effects of sitting around all day. Researchers at the University of Sydney have followed 145,000 people over the age of 45 for 9 years. They found that sitting more than 6 hours a day increased the risk of death by 4%. Fortunately, and this is part of the information provided by this study, it is quite possible to eliminate this risk by taking 30 minutes of moderate walking per day, 5 days per week[63]. The difficulty is to be able to leave your car behind to implement this recommendation. It is then necessary to move as much as possible. Do not hesitate to walk to a public transit station. The return trips made and recorded in a routine will increase your number of steps per day. Even during work, do not hesitate to move from one office to another for professional exchanges. No more using the elevators.

Alternatively, it is noted that adults with pet dogs walk much more and have more physical activity than those without dogs[64]. Although the study found that only 23% of adults walk their dogs more than 5 times a week, the results show that physical activity and the number of steps per day are 57% and 77% higher, respectively, compared to those who do not own a dog[64]. Owning and walking a dog is an opportunity to fight sedentary lifestyles and promote general well-being[65]. In the USA since 2013, a statement from the American Heart Association's has ruled on the benefits of owning a dog and its impact on physical activity, and reducing the risk of cardiovascular disease. Many experiments report that to amplify the beneficial effects of walking, it is interesting to take walks in wooded parks or in the woods. Who has never experienced this relaxing and very pleasant effect of walking, in the perfect calm of a park or a wood? It's also very good for your health and it works! Scientists have tried to understand what makes us so happy during this activity. This is a practice well known to the Japanese, who have made walking in the woods a real therapy for our health. We will talk about it in stress management.

Scheduled physical activities: Practice HIIT daily if you have little time

If you want to achieve a significant weight and abdominal circumference drop, not only should you kick out your sedentary lifestyle, but also include scheduled physical activities in your calendar. These physical activities are complementary to the other activities included in the daily routine (climbing stairs, walking, watching your diet, drinking water...). The activities programmed to achieve good results are those that fall along during the week from Monday to Friday. Saturdays can be reserved for a less intensive activity, combining sports and relaxation, such as a walk in a wooded park or in the woods. Sunday can be your day off for a rest. While respecting the number of hours required for sleep, the ideal would be to practice early morning physical activity at home. Time is an element that requires a certain anticipation, in order not to stress. To do this, allow yourself time for these activities, including time for preparation, time to do them and time to prepare for something else, such as a shower. I personally allow myself 10 minutes to prepare after waking up, 10 minutes to do exercises, 5 minutes of stretching, 5 minutes of final meditation and 5 minutes to prepare for something else. It's a total of 35 minutes, which I give myself early in the morning, for my physical activities. Without any stress. The preference for the morning is due to the feeling that at that time my body is more soothed by the calm and morning silence. It is also a good time for meditation. After a good night's sleep, getting up early is beneficial for our cardiovascular condition[66]. After a morning physical activity session, our body is better prepared and more effective in coping with the stress of the day. In my case, it is gradually that I set myself the challenge of getting up early and that in the long run has become routine. It is a process that can be natural for some people, while for others, it necessarily requires learning and adaptation phases.

These daily and morning physical activities should also include exercises that make maximum use of our muscles and joints. However, for an unaccustomed person, the pace may seem intensive at first. Programs exist on social media and smartphones; the one I recommend is HIIT for High-Intensity Interval Training to adapt to your abilities. The advantage of these exercises is that they require little space and take place in a short time (between 4 to 12 minutes). The time required to perform these exercises is shorter than that required to perform the classic and moderate cardiovascular endurance called MIIT (Moderate Intensity Interval Training). In the case of MIIT, for example, it is a matter of running for 30 minutes or more at a constant and moderate pace. It's sometimes boring, but also after a few days of sessions, the body burns far fewer calories than in the first session. The second advantage of HIIT is that it can be practiced without equipment, in order to reduce the risk of injury for a beginner. Nevertheless, it is extremely important to carry them out with great caution the first few times. Progressiveness is required. Do not engage in intensive programs or crazy sprints. Once you have mastered the technique, you will be much more comfortable and you can move on to the many variants available on your smartphone and social media apps. For these HIITs, each morning, we can start with a session of moderate HIITs per day, 3 days a week and then step up to 5 days a week.

This training combines short exercises with small recovery phases. The whole objective of HIIT is to stimulate the body's metabolism and make it active for a good part of the day. When comparing individuals subjected to 20-second intense and short exercises with a total duration of 10 minutes (HIIT), compared to those who perform 50 minutes of moderate activity, we notice that the energy expended per minute is higher in the case of HIIT. It is clear that in terms of time, and in terms of metabolic activation, if you practice a 10-minute HIIT, you will be more efficient than a person who jogs for 50 minutes. More accurate estimates confirm in other similar models that caloric expenditure is about 10 calories per minute for HIIT[67], and 7.6 calories per minute for MIIT[68]. The 10-minute HIIT will be more effective at burning fat per minute than the 50-minute jog. Nevertheless, the total number of calories expended during a 50-minute jogging session remains higher. HIIT also helps to limit muscle loss. From the age of 30, every individual begins to lose about 3% of their muscle mass every 10 years. This phenomenon is physiological and accelerates once you get to your fifties, to reach a loss of 2% per year[69]! Regardless of your age, regular use of an adapted HIIT reduces physiological muscle loss and directly fights the general ageing of the body[70]. For a person with an active life, go for an elliptical bike or treadmill rather than a conventional bike in order to waste less time. The risk of injury is reduced. The skipping rope is also interesting for those who know how to use it.

For the others, here is an example that I regularly practice that lasts 7 minutes and 50 seconds:

Example of HIIT in 12 steps[71] (to be carried out 4 to 5 times a week, with variants).

Each step is performed for 30 seconds, then followed by 10 seconds of recovery, before moving on to the next step. In the end, we arrive at a total of 7 minutes and 50 seconds. This excellent program and its variants are available in many apps and on Youtube.

1. **Jumping jacks** :

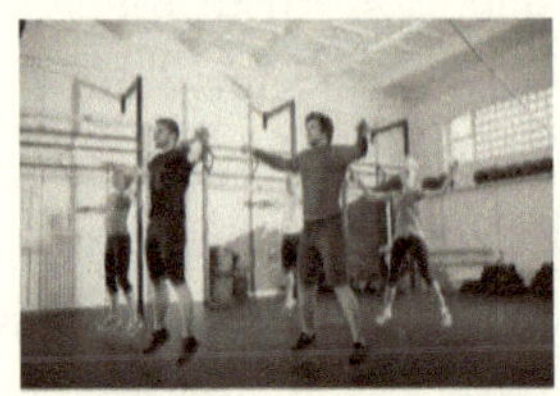

2. **Chair** :

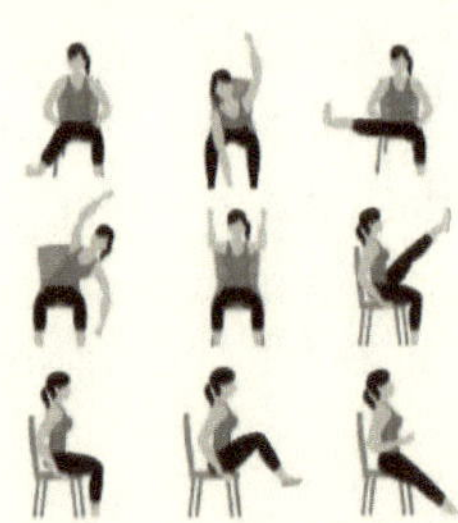

3. **Push-ups:**

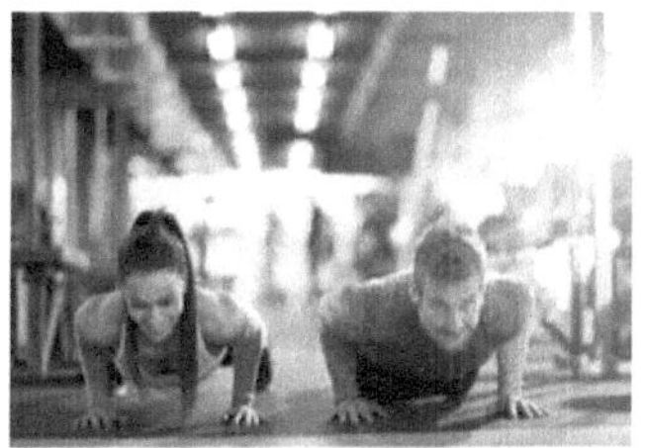

4. **Crunches :**

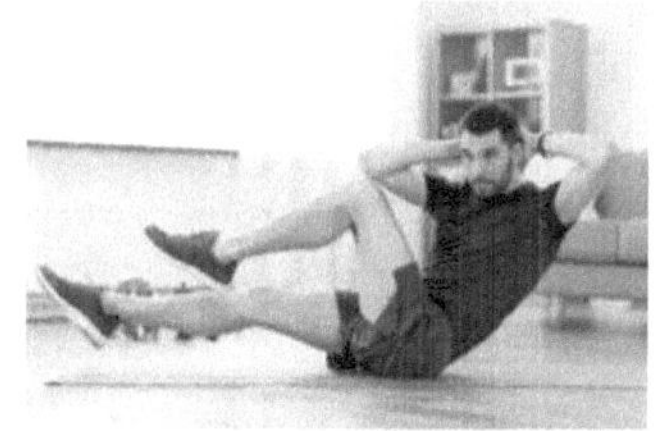

5. **Chair mount :**

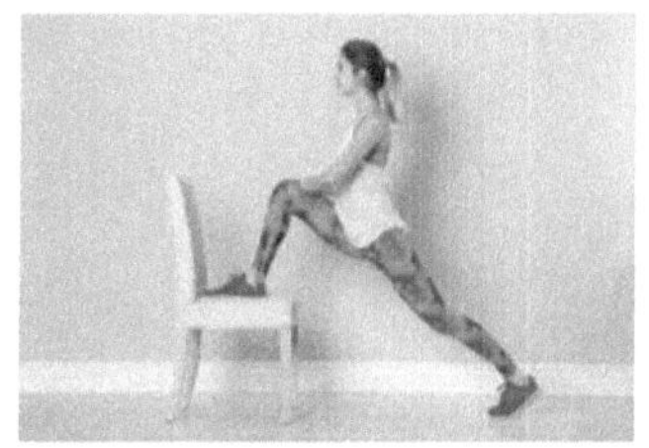

6. Squats :

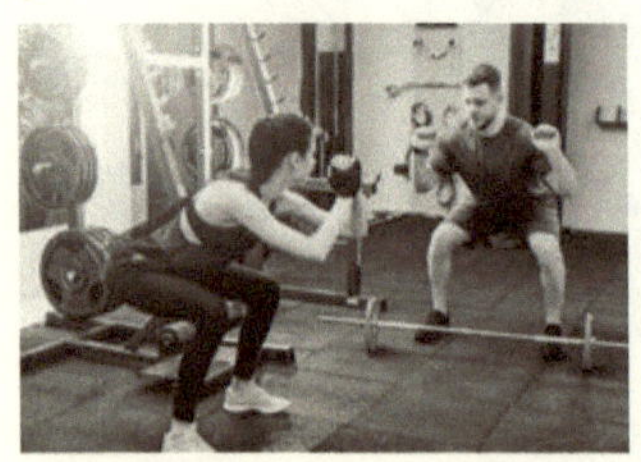

7. Chair dips :

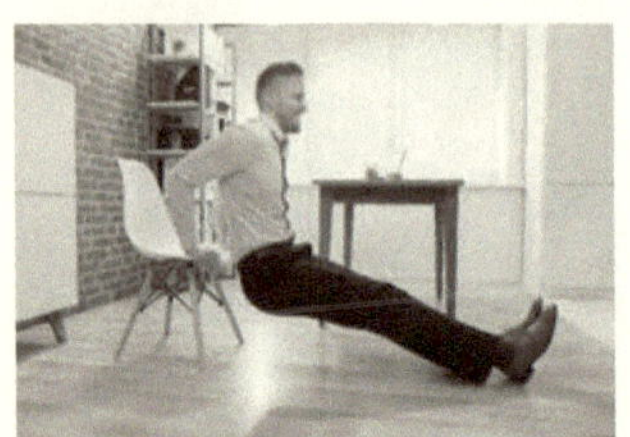

8. Plank pose :

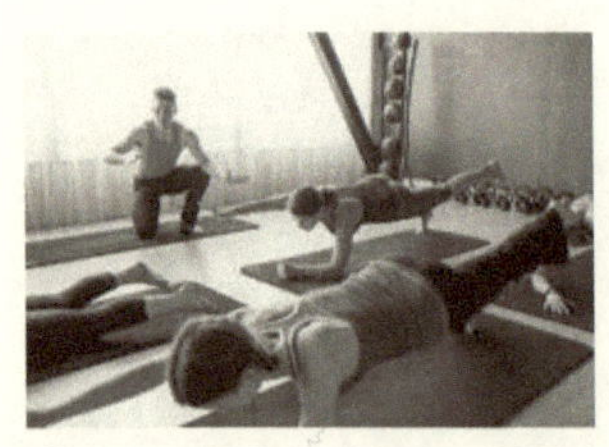

9. Running on spot :

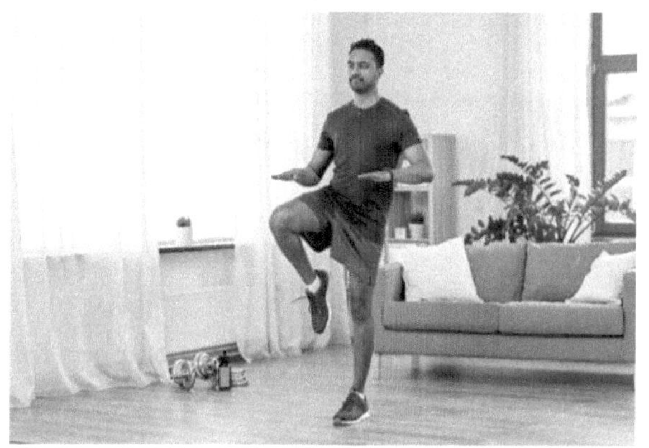

10. Lunge:

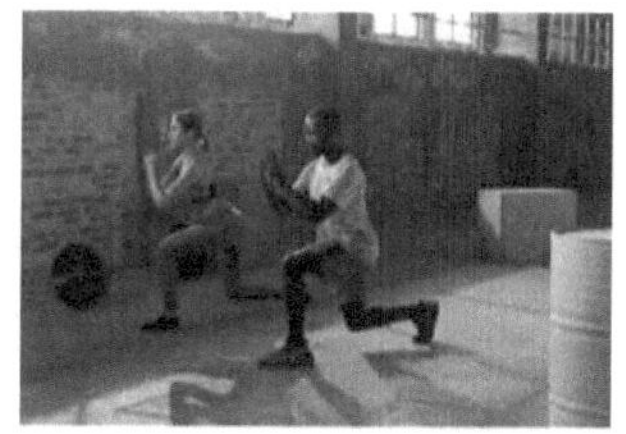

11. T push-ups :

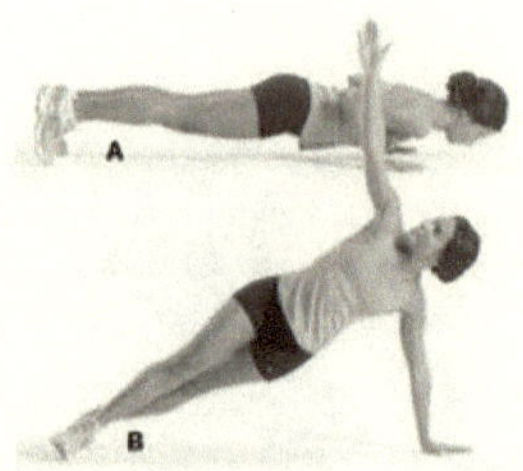

12. Lateral plank : Perform this movement for 15 seconds on each side.

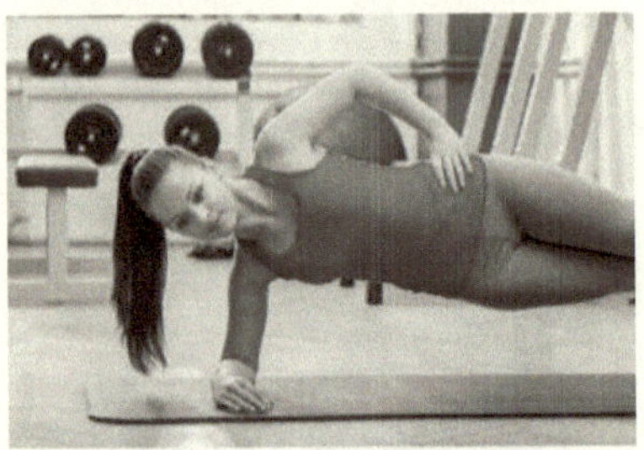

You can't rely on HITT alone to lose a lot of weight. Studies comparing HIIT and MIIT indicate a loss of fat mass in both protocols with unfortunately little impact on BMI[72]. Another Australian study goes in the same direction, and highlights the lack of impact on weight[73]. Does this mean that it is useless to expect weight loss by doing this physical activity on a regular basis? No, because on the one hand HIIT has other advantages, which can indirectly help in weight loss. Decrease in sedentary lifestyle, energy expenditure, improvement of muscle strength, psychological impact with a better quality of life[74]. In addition, regular sporting activity has many other advantages, which will be discussed later with Stress Management, Sleep Management and Chronic Disease Control. It must be part of all the strategies to be implemented. An intense activity of 10 minutes, 4 to 5 times a week, must be combined with a diet rich in fibre and vegetables to have a significant effect on weight. By combining these physical activities with others such as walking, stair climbing, stretching movements at the office and domestic activities, the objectives will necessarily be achieved.

Move like you breathe (at Work, at home...)

Any movement is better than no movement. We must make movement a real way of life. Studies go further and advise to move and oscillate your legs or feet discreetly under the desk. In other words, stay seated and move your legs as soon as you can! This is one of the solutions for those who work many hours sitting down. The observation of the cardiac and energetic activity of workers was studied in successive positions, sitting, standing, and sitting with legs moving. It is clear from this that working seated by moving the legs allows a higher energy expenditure than working standing or sitting without moving the legs[75].

Another solution to be promoted at work is the generalization of seats that can alternate sitting and standing positions. Working standing up makes us spend 0.15 calories per minute. In one day of work, it represents more than 60 calories expended[76]. It's good for losing weight, but in the long term. Working upright helps to set the body in motion. There is strengthening of our muscular capacities, maintenance of good circulation. We are thus constantly in motion, and the energy expenditure is higher than that of the sitting position. At first, this practice raised some concerns[77]. Even the Wall Street Journal advised against standing for long periods of time[78]. It has been found, for example, that people in good health complain of back pain after two hours of standing work[79]. To avoid this back pain, it is advisable to alternate with the sitting position, while moving as much as possible. Over a one-hour period, you can sit for 40 minutes and stand for 16 minutes. The remaining 4 minutes should be used for discreet stretching. The layout of the office elements can also be optimized. To do this, the layout of the work equipment must encourage people to walk as little as possible. It is advisable to have the printer away from the office or to have toilets on the first floor, which means taking the stairs to get there.

Moving must also be done at home. Be more active in everyday life. Don't hesitate to do more housework and enjoy doing it. It is a considerable way to keep in shape. You need to fight sedentary lifestyles by all means. Norwegian scientists have been working to understand the impact of household activities on our health[80]. For this purpose, they followed for 6 years, more than 30,000 individuals carrying devices, which allow them to be classified into different groups, according to their level of activity. The researchers found that physical activity, regardless of its intensity, reduces the risk of early death. The risk of death can be reduced by up to 15% when moderate domestic activities reach 5 hours per day. For the very active, the reduction can reach 70%! And the study also provides a very interesting clarification: the beneficial effect begins as soon as a minimum of 24 minutes of household tasks are performed. Thus cooking, gardening, actively participating in the tidying up and maintenance of the house is widely recommended to keep in good shape. These recommendations are in line with the 150 minutes of moderate activity recommended by the World Health Organization.

Did you know? To keep your spirits up, there's nothing better than taking advantage of the changing seasons to review your living space. It is not necessarily a matter of spending many hours on it, but of making minimal changes to brighten up your living space. For example, you can focus on a single part, and redo the painting: Color change, controlled time and satisfaction are guaranteed. This change will give you the opportunity to go to a DIY store, get the necessary equipment, and discover the latest ideas in the field of painting. Redesigning your interior with minimal modifications is inspired by the philosophy of Feng Shui, an ancestral Chinese practice. Minor changes in materials, colours, lighting, odours or bed orientation, for example, can sometimes have a significant impact on quality of life.

Gradually go for dark chocolate

Dark chocolate has qualities that can help to avoid snacking. We all experience these moments of stress or intense activity, which push us in search of a comforting food. At these precise moments, dark chocolate can replace most of the products that make us fat. Dark chocolate is a real storage warehouse for compounds called flavonoids. These flavonoids have very interesting properties that protect against cellular ageing. By unit weight, dark chocolate contains more flavonoids than products known to contain flavonoids such as red wine, black tea, apples or cranberry juice[81].

On a sample of 20 people, 40 g of dark chocolate with 70% cocoa, proved to be an excellent appetite suppressant after 4 weeks[82]. In another study, an intake of 30 g of dark chocolate with 85% cocoa resulted in a decrease in appetite[83]. For the caloric aspect, the number of calories ingested, per day, is significantly lower, compared to milk chocolate[84]. By consuming more than 70% of dark chocolate, the total number of calories consumed daily is 120 calories less, with an effect on immediate satiety. The reduction in appetite is thought to be the result of a proliferation of good bacteria, namely lactobacilli and bifodobacteria, and the decrease in bad bacteria, such as clostridium, due to the flavoinoid compounds in dark chocolate[85]. For my part, it is interesting, when looking for a hunger suppressant effect, to start with dark chocolate at least 80% of the time and limit yourself to 2 squares of dark chocolate or 20 grams per day. There is no disadvantage, if a person wants to switch to a dark chocolate with 90% cocoa that has a more bitter taste. The most important thing is to go gradually to get the brain used to the special taste of dark chocolate.

Would you really lose weight by fasting?

Fasting is a way of dieting that can help you lose weight. This involves alternating more or less long periods of fasting with periods of food intake. Intermittent fasting is the most common form, compared to strict fasting, which is a food deprivation over several days. Most of the time, intermittent fasting involves a period of food deprivation of 16 to 48 hours, or cyclically every other day, while avoiding or limiting caloric intake over this period[86]. Different intermittent fasting plans are proposed, and the results on weight loss are variable.

For example, over 2 days of the week, caloric intake is reduced by about 75%. The individual will then consume between 500 and 600 calories over the 2 days of diet. Over the other 5 days, the food is reintroduced in a normal way, without excess. This diet makes it possible to lose weight in the long term. This is the 5:2 diet. In a study involving 115 individuals, this type of fasting (2 days of fasting with 70% caloric restriction with 40 gr of carbohydrates) was compared to a 7-day low-calorie Mediterranean diet. The results showed that the intermittent fasting of 2 days has a more marked effect on weight reduction[87]. These results are due to the fact that individuals prefer the 2-day intermittent fasting to a diet that should last one week. In addition, the possibility of choosing the 2 days of the week makes it easier to accept this plan.

Intermittent fasting over 2 days seems to be the best compromise. This diet can be followed every other day or over a shorter period of 12 or 16 hours. When I practice it, I prefer to fast from 8 p.m. to 12 p.m. the next day, which is like eating early in the evening and skipping breakfast and then eating at 12 noon.

STRESS

If there is one thing that has a significant impact on the overall quality of our lives, it's stress. Worldwide, the criteria for defining stress are variable, and depend on socio-cultural habits. While in some countries stress can be defined by the feeling of a working day, in another country it can be defined by the availability of food. It is estimated, through a Gallup Institute survey, that more than 33% of people worldwide consider themselves stressed, and that the United States is among the top 10 countries where people report being stressed[88]. Acute stress, which stimulates us at a specific moment, is not the most harmful. It is the one that settles in and has a lasting impact on our days, which is the most to be feared. In fact, it is the way of life we are faced with that is at the heart of the problem. For reasons that seem obvious to us and that are obvious to us, we must respect a schedule from the morning, eat breakfast, go to work in as little time as possible, and keep a full day between the demands of work and personal life. In recent years, new technologies, and especially smartphones, have been added to this way of life. All this to such an extent that today it is extremely difficult not to own a smartphone. This permanent race eventually triggers harmful and devastating effects on our body.

Permanent stress triggers autoimmune diseases

Autoimmune diseases are diseases that occur when the body's immune system eliminates normal body components. It is a dysfunction that can lead to diseases such as Crohn's disease, multiple sclerosis or rheumatoid arthritis. Several factors can trigger autoimmune disease. Stress is one of these elements. In a Swedish study, individuals with psychiatric problems, who were subjected to emotional and prolonged stress, were followed for 10 years[89]. During the 10 years, all cases of new autoimmune diseases were recorded. The researchers noted that compared to individuals without stress, those exposed to permanent stress had a 46% higher risk of developing an autoimmune disease.

This study confirms what has been observed in Vietnam War veterans undergoing post-traumatic stress[92] [93]. The type of diseases triggered by permanent stress is variable. In the case of individuals with psychiatric illnesses, they get celiac disease, an intolerance to gluten absorption, as a majority, while in the case of veterans, it is rheumatoid arthritis. Thus, prolonged stress can trigger and completely deregulate hormones in our body[94]. In the context of post-traumatic stress (see box), interleukins and interferons are also involved[95]. Worse still, perceived stress can lead to a relapse of autoimmune diseases, for people considered cured for certain diseases. This was noted in 13 Japanese hospitals, where there was a significant increase in hemorrhagic recto-colitis relapses after earthquakes[96].

Permanent stress evolves into anxiety, and affects brain capacity.

In some situations, we may feel very worried. It is an impression of inner tension or imminent danger. We don't feel well. Generally, this situation occurs when, for example, a lack of time, knowledge or financial resources means that we do not feel that we match up to the objectives we have set for ourselves. This may include, for example, the organisation of an exceptional trip, working conditions or the organisation of our weekly planning. It is a recurrent phenomenon, to which we are regularly subjected, and which disturbs our focus for everyday life. This phenomenon, when it is not excessive, is normal, and is intended to allow us to adapt, according to the various situations we face. When this phenomenon becomes chronic, i.e. with permanent stress, it will gradually evolve into a state of anxiety, and can impact our overall health. Studies have shown that women exposed to stress are twice as affected by anxiety as men[97]. Similarly, the effect of moderate and permanent stress induces mood disorders, and a state of depression. Several evaluations using different sources of stress have shown that individuals under stress eventually develop negative emotions and cardiovascular disturbances[98]. Imaging and facial analysis techniques have confirmed that, under the influence of permanent stress, individuals eventually become angry and anxious[99] [100]. Similarly, chronic stress causes mood swings and depression[101]. This is due to the permanence of a high cortisol level, which alters many brain functions, and leads to sleep disorders[102]. In any individual, the effects of stress on the body begin from the prenatal period and last a lifetime. The impact on brain function will depend on the duration of exposure to stress[103]. The time of exposure to stress affects the weight of the brain, and makes it atrophic[104]. Thus, long-term stress is particularly harmful to both the functioning and structure of the brain.

In a study involving a sample of more than 2000 individuals, whose morning cortisol levels were regularly monitored, researchers used imaging techniques to establish a link between cortisol level and brain volume. High cortisol levels are found in most individuals with both small brain volume and impaired brain function[105]. Several studies follow the same line, concluding that chronic stress destroys brain cells over time[106][107].

Stress and junk food

Stress can increase the risk of chronic diseases through some bad daily habits. A person who is very often exposed to a particular stress will develop certain habits to better resist this stress: coffee, alcohol, cigarettes or sweet and fatty foods. The link between alcohol consumption and stress is known[108]. In 2014, the Gallup Institute's report on stress reported that 49% of Americans consume at least once a week a very poor quality and calorie-rich diet in response to stress[109]. This phenomenon is dependent on two hormones, cortisol and ghrelin. Following stress, it is noticed that 20 to 30 minutes after a release of cortisol in the blood, the appetite is stimulated, accompanied by a strong desire for snacking with an attraction for foods such as fries, chips, biscuits, popcorn and donuts[110]. Stimuli triggering high cortisol levels have confirmed this desire to eat particularly sweet foods[111].

Ghrelin, a digestive hormone, is considered the hunger hormone because its level is high before meals, and decreases as soon as the stomach is full. Under the effect of acute stress, its blood level is significantly increased[112]. Researchers believe that these fluctuations are also involved in the consumption of caloric foods with low nutritional value[113]. Apart from these hormones, psychological conditions would also explain the link between stress and junk food. Anxiety and depression generated by stress are conditions that lead to the search for foods high in sugar and fat[114 115], or even to a large number of meals[116].

Stress and some cancers

A link has always been suspected between stress and certain cancers. Patients report permanent or intense stress, which may have triggered their cancer. Inflammatory mechanisms triggered by stress are believed to be involved in the genesis of some cancers. This link has been confirmed for some breast cancers. Intense stress of more than one month leads to the development of rapidly growing cancer cells[117]. The researchers explain that the adrenaline secreted under stress activates the proliferation of cancer cells.

In 2018, a link between psychological stress and breast cancer incidence was established after follow-up of women with breast cancer in some companies[118]. Nevertheless, doubts remain, and some studies conclude that the link between cancer and stress is the result of a perception of high stress, associated with cancer risk[119]. Regarding colorectal cancer, while a link has been established with rectal cancer, none has been established with colon cancer[120]. Researchers in Munich believe that a disturbance of the intestinal flora under stress would cause tumours only in the colon. In this case, it is not the stress experienced during the individual's life that would be the cause, but the impact of this stress on the microbiota[121]. As we can see, stress and its effects on cancer have not yet revealed all their secrets. However, in the absence of clear data, it is prudent not to be overwhelmed by stress, and to promote solutions to reduce their impact.

Chronic stress accelerates cell aging

Cellular aging is one of the harmful and insidious effects of chronic stress on our body. Many studies explain that the cardiovascular effects, and the cancers observed, are actually the consequences of a more complicated phenomenon, called oxidative stress. Physiologically, cell ageing involves the shortening of part of the DNA, known as telomeres, and the grafting of methyl-type chemical groups onto the DNA. Under the effect of stress, telomeres are shortened and the cells age. It is clearly observed that stressed mothers who care for a chronically ill child on a daily basis have shortened telomeres. The most stressed women are said to have aged more than 9 to 17 years, compared to those who are not stressed[122]. The shortening of telomers due to oxidative stress has also been observed in children aged 3 to 15 exposed to stress, such as domestic violence, disappearances or institutionalization. There is even an observed association between mothers with severe depression and the length of children's telomeres[123]. In adult individuals, a cumulative effect of stress over the entire lifespan has an impact on the length of telomeres. The more stressed you are, the shorter the telomeres get. Even the cumulative effects of stress during childhood have a significant impact on the length of telomeres[124].

Stress is involved in cardiovascular disease

An individual under permanent stress increases their risk of cardiovascular disease by 64% [125]. And this, no matter the origin of the stress! The manifestations of this type of chronic stress begin within the first 6 to 12 months after the onset of the stressful event. It is in individuals under 50 years of age that the effects are particularly pronounced. Similarly, acute stress can have a disastrous effect on the heart. It was noted during the July 2006 World Cup matches in Germany that heart attacks were multiplied by 4, among individuals who had already had heart problems, and by 2 among people who did not have such problems[126]. A similar phenomenon was observed in 2011 during the earthquakes in Japan, where the number of sudden deaths was twice as high as in previous years[127]. Sudden stress can even temporarily modify the cardiac morphology, and more precisely the left ventricle, following intense emotional stress. It's called "broken heart syndrome" or tako-tsubo. On the other hand, permanent stress can lead to anxiety and other much more serious disorders. To illustrate the link between stress and cardiovascular impact, in 1974, Roseman and Friedman, two cardiologists, described the typical case of personality A, characterized by an intensive daily rhythm, which is constantly seeking high professional efficiency[128]. This typical profile, subjected to this permanent stress, has a risk of cardiovascular diseases multiplied by 2, compared to a normal subject. In a study published in 2017, researchers showed that chronic stress involves the activity of the brain's tonsil, which emits pro-inflammatory signals responsible for cardiovascular events[129]. When we are under constant stress, our brain, through the tonsil, emits signals that are very harmful to the heart and arteries.

Did you know? The tonsil of the brain (not to be confused with that of the throat), is a structure with a kernel shape, and located just in front of the hippocampus. It plays a role in managing our emotions, fear and anxiety. When both tonsils of the brain are damaged, the patient no longer feels fear or pleasure.

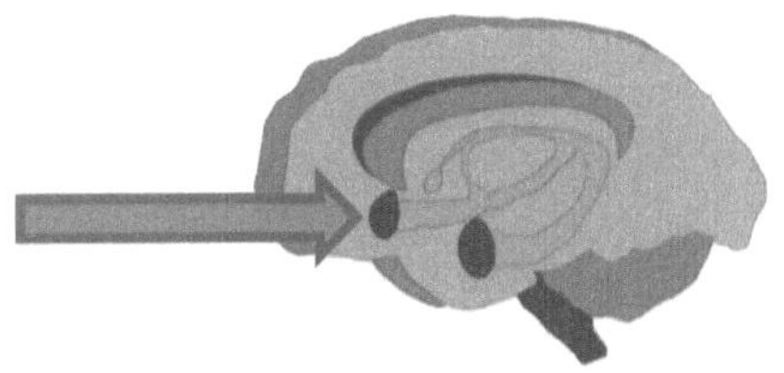

Stress causes sleep disorders and alters the hippocampus.

Who has never experienced a sleep disorder during acute stress? Stress has a direct impact on this essential element of our well-being. Acute stress can lead to a hard time falling asleep, or alter the quality of sleep, for example, by reducing the duration of sleep. Sleep disorders will generate anxiety, and all this will lead to a vicious circle. This is especially the case of chronic stress, which will lead to a gradual increase in cortisol levels in the blood. This condition will eventually lead to nocturnal awakenings, which in turn will lead to cortisol stimulation.

Did you know? The hippocampus is a part of the brain. It plays an important role in the processes of memorization, attention, and perception of space. Like the tonsil of the brain, its volume is reduced during chronic stress.

In Alzheimer's disease, for example, the hippocampus is one of the parts of the brain that is affected early. Its involvement in depression has been the subject of much research. For a long time, it was recognized that the renewal of neurons is an impossible phenomenon, it has been demonstrated, by staining techniques, that the hippocampus is capable of producing new neurons, in adults.

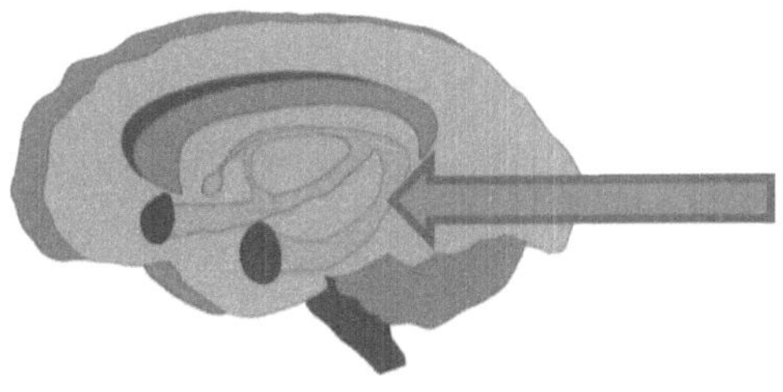

These chronic disorders will lead to depression and anxiety [130]. If depression and anxiety are chronic, the risk of a change in brain capacity, and more specifically atrophy of the hippocampus, is increased [104].

Physical activity reduces stress and its effects on the brain

So what is the solution? We are inadvertently confronted with stress and we need to overcome it. Solutions do exist. It is well known that all newspapers and websites promote sport as a stress relief measure. We have already experienced that physical activity is an excellent way to lose weight, especially when diet is controlled. Being physically active and regular, reduces the effects of daily stress. Several rigorous studies have demonstrated the effectiveness of physical activity in improving mental state and quality of life. In an Australian study, individuals who did not exercise at all, and who were encouraged to exercise for 20 minutes, 3 times a week, had a significant improvement in their mental health and more specifically in anxiety, depression and stress, with a strong impact on quality of life[131]. Other studies, carried out under the same conditions, show similar results considered spectacular [132]. Depression, one of the consequences of stress, is reduced by 26%, and can even reach 68% in joggers[133]. These results are particularly interesting, compared to antidepressants whose overall efficacy is estimated at 50%, with all possible side effects[134]. Generally speaking, it is established that physical activity can reduce intense stress by 78%, and by 62% for moderate stress, as soon as caloric expenditure reaches 300 calories per day.

The explanation is that physical exercise reduces acute and chronic stress by influencing cardiac physiology. Individuals who engage in regular physical activity have a resting blood pressure that is significantly lower than those who are less active[135]. Moderate or strenuous activity reduces the effects of stress on blood pressure, with a reduction in adrenergic discharge. Better still, physical activity affects the plasticity of the brain, through the formation of new blood vessels. By stimulating this training, physical exercise maintains the birth of new neurons, with the consequence of preventive action, which reduces the decrease in the volume of the hippocampus[136]. As shown in the Australian study, 20 minutes of daily physical activity 3 times a week is enough to have a significant effect on stress and its brain consequences. All we have to do now is put it into practice and I assure you it works.

Relax and practice music therapy

Frequently our body gives us signals that it is necessary to appease it. One of the measures to fight stress is to take your time to relax. This time is personal time, which must be spent regularly. The most important thing is to make a regular cut. It can even be integrated into your daily lifestyle. There are many examples. For example, you can go to a library and browse magazines. You can play a musical instrument that you love very much. Or, for those who live in countries with cold climates, spend a morning in resorts equipped with swimming pools, saunas and massage rooms. For those who are in warmer countries, do not hesitate to go to the pool that cools the body, or play under a tree in group games. This break reduces by one notch all the tension that an individual can accumulate over a certain period of time. It is extremely important to do what you love, in a suitable environment that allows for a real break. Again, this is a moment for yourself.

Listening to music you like is a simple and enjoyable way to relax. This effect can reduce stress in a very significant way! In Paris, for example, some hospitals make use of instruments and musicians in pre-anaesthesia rooms for children to accompany them to the operating room. A German study, analyzing the effect of music on stressed individuals, showed a reduction in the perception of stress, accompanied by a significant decrease in cortisol. The authors of the study pointed out that the anti-stress effect of music is all the stronger when it is known as relaxing music[137]. Thus, to reduce stress, listening to Wolfgang Amadeus Mozart or Richard Strauss for 25 minutes a day is an excellent way to lower blood pressure and cortisol levels[138].

Laughter and friendliness reduce stress

Try a short experiment when you are alone: focus and remember a past event that made you laugh. You will feel for a short while that your mood will shift to something more positive that improves your stress. If possible, and provided you have good relationships, repeat this experience later, but this time with someone with whom you have shared a moment of laughter in the past about a particular event. If, despite the passage of time, the person remembers this mad laughter, and it takes you back into a mad laughter, you will feel the joys of laughter and friendliness. Laughter heals and reduces our stress. Cardiologists are aware of this. As kids, we laughed 400 times a day, when we grew up, that number dropped to 10 a day. The health benefits of laughter were first reported by Norman Cousins, an American journalist with a strong medical culture[139]. In 1964, when he was hospitalized for ankylosing spondylitis, he took the decision to leave the hospital, and to stay in a hotel and take care of himself with vitamin C. He was diagnosed with ankylosing spondylitis. To break with the isolation, he bought comic films, and it is with surprise that he saw that the madman laughed to relieve his pain. Decades later, science provides tools to understand the involvement of endorphins and, certainly other anti-inflammatory mediators, in the relief of Norman Cousins. Using laughter to relieve stress is undoubtedly the most economical way: it costs nothing, can be done over short and repeated periods of time. It is recognized that the immediate effect of laughter is just as effective on stress as physical activity and music[140]. Genuine laughter, which is spontaneous laughter, has an extremely beneficial effect on mood. This type of spontaneous laughter reduces cortisol levels by more than 50%

after watching a 60-minute comedy film[141]. But, it is possible to cause laughter, to benefit from these effects on stress. This is the case, for example, for yoga and group relaxation sessions. This type of approach has also shown important results on mood improvement[142]. Short-term laughter experiences are very effective[143], each person can set up conditions that allow them to regularly remember situations that provoke laughter. The ideal would be, for example, to listen to short extracts of comic stories, lasting 5 minutes twice a day and in a good mood. And remember this trick: keep in mind a particular event that has always made you laugh. In case of stress, or anger-type mood swings, think about this event. It will help you.

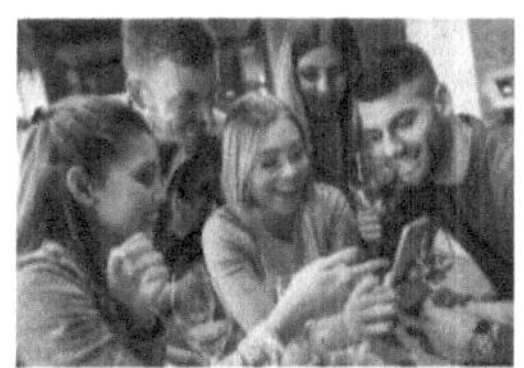

Forest walking is an anti-stress activity

I had recommended walking for weight management, and if possible in the woods, or in a wooded park, for those who live in large cities. It is recommended to ensure safe conditions for this type of activity, as it requires walking in areas where there is little traffic, and preferably at times when the calm would be perfect. This practice has its origins in the life of Henry David Thoreau, philosopher and naturalist, who wrote "Walden or Life in the Woods", a true reflection on the economy, nature and simple life led away from society. He spent years observing the changing seasons, fauna and flora. He was so fascinated by nature that he called for her respect. At the time, of course, evidence of nature's impact on our well-being was not on the agenda. Similarities can be observed among the Japanese people, who have a long tradition of walking in the forests to calm down. This is what is known as the "Japanese Walk". For the Japanese, it is a real physical and psychological immersion in the forest in order to benefit from nature's therapeutic assets, while showing great respect for it. Walking in the forest, to get rid of all the stress buried in the depths of our being. In the 1980s, inspired by the Shinto religion, which has a great respect for nature, the Japanese government promoted the "Shinrin-yoku" or forest bath to recharge its batteries in the heart of nature. The practice consists of walking in the forest, taking the time to capture the sounds that prevail there, looking at the tops of the trees. You can walk along the trails provided for this purpose, or just sit on a bench in a wooded park and contemplate nature for 20 to 30 minutes. For cold regions, it is essential to protect yourself well. In an experiment conducted in 24 Japanese forests, researchers analyzed the impact of "Shinrin-yoku" on our overall health[144]. Biological variables, such as cortisol levels, blood pressure, heart rate and pulse rate, were analyzed on a sample of 280 individuals, walking alternately for 30 minutes in the forest or in the city. The results showed that, compared to walking in the city, walking in the forest reduces cortisol levels, lowers heart rate, lowers blood pressure, increases parasympathetic nerve activity, and low adrenergic activity. We deduce that a 30-minute walk in the forest, or in a wooded park, reduces the secretion of cortisol and adrenaline, which is very important for reducing stress. According to Professor Qing Li's research, natural killer cells (NK) of the immune system, before and after exposure to essential oils from wood, allow our body to react more vigorously to all external attacks[145]. Forest air releases essential oils called phytoncides, which improve the immune system's function. Even if the link between stress and phytoncids has yet to be understood, everyone agrees that it is extremely relaxing to take a 30-minute break in a park. Additional evidence has been reported to demonstrate the effectiveness of walking on individuals living in urban areas and walking in tree-lined parks[146]. Scientists from the University of Michigan followed 36 subjects living in urban areas for two months. Three times a week, they had to spend 10 minutes or more in contact with nature, and their salivary cortisol level was analyzed. The results showed that a daily break of 20 to 30 minutes allowed a significant reduction in cortisol levels.

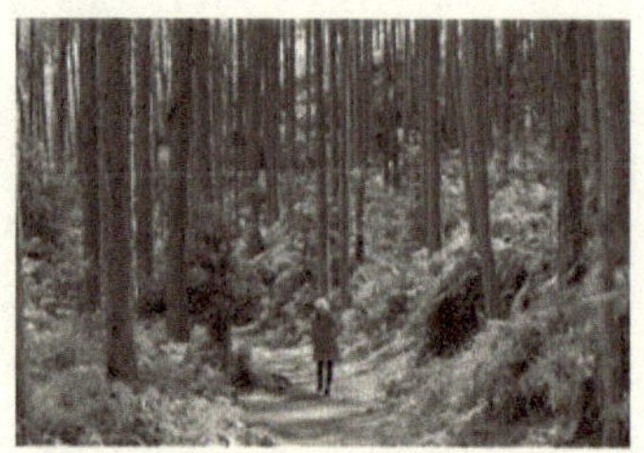

Practice regular meditation for your brain functions

It is useful to allow yourself time to meditate. Meditation brings serenity and clarity. It is a state of great concentration of the mind to deepen the thinking about oneself. It goes beyond relaxation. It is a necessary moment for a total disconnection from the disturbances of life. Meditation is not a difficult task. It requires a quiet place, where you are not likely to be disturbed. You can meditate in your room, in a park or in a garden, or even by listening to appropriate music. I have a preference for a short meditation after the morning physical exercises. It is a quiet time when during the beautiful seasons, you can have the opportunity to observe the sunrise. Concerning the position, there is no absolute position to adopt. The lotus position is one of many, but it can give a beginner more confidence. A simple chair or a comfortable armchair may suffice. The position must be comfortable and allow breathing movements to be performed according to our wishes. The arms can be placed on the thighs, knees along the body... and close your eyes.

It is not a question of seeking to reach the spiritual level of the great masters of meditation, but of finding a balance that leads you to focus your thoughts. The act of meditation itself is to focus on an imaginary object in your mind, or to make a void in your mind, or to leave thoughts, feelings and emotions as time goes by, and not to judge them as good or bad. Listen to your breathing with your eyes closed.

Another technique is to practice "mindfulness" which consists in concentrating on your sensations, your breathing, your emotions, your present thoughts, and to avoid worrying about your past or future anxieties. It is important to note that there are several meditation techniques, with quite different principles.

Did you know? Mindfulness-based stress reduction (MBSR) is a meditation technique developed at the University of Massachusetts Medical Center in the 1970s by Professor Jon Kabat-Zinn. The principle is to focus attention on the present moment, which promotes full self-awareness. To understand, it is enough to realize, what sometimes happens to us when we take a bus from one destination A to another destination B, and when we arrive, we do not remember any event seen on the journey, or even certain stages of the journey. We were not aware of all the events around us during this journey. Where was our mind then? Certainly open to anxious thoughts. Through learning with mindfulness, the individual learns to regulate his emotions and thoughts, and to refocus on himself.

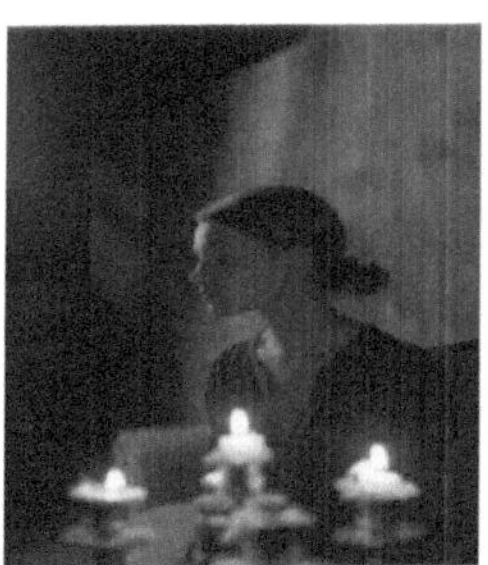

Meditation helps to achieve mental balance, and to be less subject to mood fluctuations. It helps us to limit the negative effects of stress, and strengthens our ability to control events that happen to us. Although subject to some doubt, several studies have shown that meditation is an excellent way to manage anxious people. In an analysis of studies collecting a total of 2466 observations on anxiety, meditation is as effective as the usual recognized techniques (medication, physical activity, music therapy...) after 6 to 12 weeks of sessions[147]. Even in the case of post-traumatic stress disorder, meditation was better than usual therapies. Out of a sample of 203 soldiers suffering from post-traumatic stress disorder, and benefiting from either 20 minutes of meditation or usual therapy daily, 61% of those who received meditation saw their symptoms improve, while only 42% of those who received usual therapy saw their symptoms improve[148]. Similarly, compared to the usual therapy, a high proportion of soldiers who received meditation agreed to complete it because they found it easier to follow. In general, meditation is a solution for attention disorders, or in case of hyperactivity. An individual assails with feelings of sadness, despair, or even loss of motivation, can gradually, through meditation, control his state and find emotional balance. The effectiveness of meditation has even been compared to the use of antidepressant medications[149]. Both treatments were positive for depression and equally effective. Meditation can be an alternative for people wishing to take antidepressants, and medications to treat anxiety. To maximize the chances of success, meditation sessions should last between 8 and 12 weeks. It is a regular practice, which has an activity on brain function. Over time, there is a reorganization of the activity of the brain circuits that regulate attention and emotions. Imaging techniques show that after 8 weeks of meditation, there is a change in brain structures, with grey matter more concentrated in the hippocampus[150] and a better connection of the brain amygdala with the prefrontal cortex. The prefrontal cortex is a part of the brain involved in decision-making, analyzing complex situations and in the ability to step back, keep cool and organize the strategies necessary to deal with a problem[152].

All these modifications explain the effectiveness of mindfulness meditation on emotions[151].

Meditation is ultimately about stimulating the birth of new neural connections that help us cope with stress.

Reduce your mental workload: List your needs for the next day before going to bed, prioritize and delegate

Reduce your stress by prioritizing the list of certain tasks you are used to doing on a regular basis. If you are used to doing certain things over the course of a week, such as shopping or going to get fuel, try to group them together. Accept the help of a close person or do not hesitate to ask for help to unburden yourself as soon as possible. Learn to keep the unexpected in perspective and then manage them in a calm environment. By introducing this habit, you will eventually simplify your daily routine and free up time for yourself.

SLEEPING

Sleep is an essential element for our body. It allows it to be regenerated and all the tension accumulated during a day of activity to be relieved. The cells that make up our organs are continuously being renewed: 20 billion of our cells die and are replaced every day and this renewal process takes place mainly during sleep. An adult human being needs 7 to 9 hours of sleep per day to fully regenerate his or her body[153]. Some individuals called "short sleepers" are content with about 6 hours of sleep, while others called "long sleepers" would rather need 10 hours. The majority of individuals who sleep less than 7 hours per night, are more likely to be exposed to the adverse effects of sleep deprivation and the cumulative long-term results impact not so positively on their life expectancy.

The development of new technologies and the demands of modern life are new elements that take precedence over the hours spent sleeping. In Western countries, for example, sleep deprivation affects 20 to 30% of the population[154] [155] [156] and at the national level, the impact on the economy is significant. For example, studies estimate the financial cost of insomnia to be $45 billion per year for Australia[157]. For the United States, at 400 billion per year[158].

> Did you know? Hypnotics are drugs that help you fall asleep. They should not be mistaken for anxiolytics, which are drugs that fight anxiety. Hypnotics and anxiolytics act on the central nervous system, which is why they are considered in medical jargon as psychotropic drugs. Hypnotics are taken in the evening at bedtime and generally require 60 to 90 minutes to induce sleep, while anxiolytics are taken between one and three times a day. Anxiolytics can also induce sleep but less effectively. Long-term use, i.e. more than 3 months of these drugs, leads to dependence. They are also suspected as a risk factor for Alzheimer's disease

Sadly, over the past few decades, the response to sleep deprivation has been to take sleeping pills, these drugs being designed to make it easier to fall asleep. It is common in Western countries to find that the number of people using these drugs can reach alarming proportions. In the United States, while the rate among 18-35 year olds is 15%, it rises to 31% among those over 65 years[159][160]. In Europe and among people over 80 years old,

94

the intake of hypnotics differs according to medical practices and ranges from 8% among Finns to 48% among the Dutch. These drugs are not free of acute side effects and can in no way be used to solve sleep-related problems. It is essential to understand that over time and age, the quality and rhythm of sleep changes in humans. Sleep begins to gradually split up from the age of 50 and people sleep less well after 80, with waking up during the night while the need for a number of hours of sleep remains at around 7 hours[161].

Did you know? Sleep is made up of:

1) An awakening phase

2) Slow sleep itself divided into 3 phases: falling asleep, light slow sleep, deep slow sleep. This phase is necessary for the physical recovery of the individual.

3) REM sleep, named after the rapid eye movements that occur during this phase (this sleep is called REM sleep because the individual presents both signs of very deep sleep and signs of awakening). It allows psychic recovery and it is the time of dreams and nightmares.

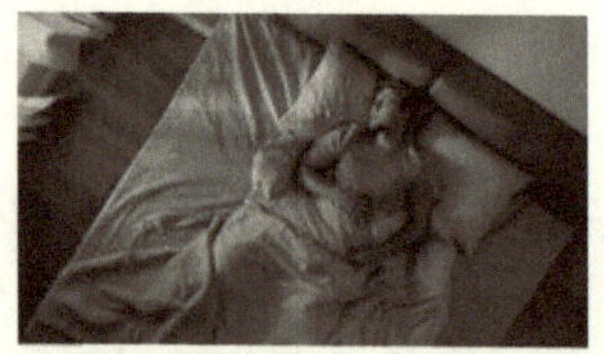

Besides, the possible disruption related to age, under professional and family constraints, hyperactivity, the omnipresence of screens, noise pollution, and stress, a disruption of sleep phases quickly occurred! It then becomes extremely complex to respect the 7 to 9 hours of sleep per night. As a result, we are now starting to accumulate sleep debt that threatens our overall well-being and its long-term sustainability. What are the real risks of accumulating sleep debt?

Lack of sleep can lead to obesity

Who has never felt after a night of very short sleep, the need to eat the next day, hot croissants and high-calorie dishes? Scientists point to a very close link between sleep deprivation and obesity. The data are accurate: It is mainly individuals sleeping less than 6 hours per night that would be most affected. And in the long term, accumulating these sleep debts can simply lead to obesity. When an individual gets into the habit of sleeping very little, he or she ends up having a clear preference for fatty and sweet dishes when waking up[162]. An analysis of several studies involving more than 600,000 young and adult individuals shows that the risk of obesity is higher among individuals with low sleep hours[163]. If you don't get enough sleep, you will automatically have a preference for fatty and sweet foods. But even more importantly, the stress caused by sleep debt stimulates a very complex system called the endocannabinoid system, whose main role is to restore the body to its perfect balance by absorbing many calories. This system is 33% more stimulated after a poor quality night and remains high until about 9pm the next day instead of decreasing fairly quickly[162].

We have already mentioned the involvement of ghrelin[113]. The lack of sleep activates the production of this hormone, which increases its rate with the consequence of a more pronounced feeling of hunger. And researchers are still very accurate in estimating that an individual will absorb an additional 385 calories to compensate for a short night's[158]. In short, not getting enough sleep greatly increases the risk of getting fatter.

Lack of sleep is a risk factor for type 2 diabetes

Newspapers and magazines don't mention it much, but a lack of sleep can lead to type 2 diabetes. At first glance, the connection does not seem at all obvious. Various studies suggest that lack of sleep leads to hormonal imbalance that can lead to type 2 diabetes in the long term. By following a group of men with sleep problems for 15 years, the researchers established the link between type 2 diabetes and sleep[163 164]. They noticed that those who sleep less than 6 hours a night are twice as likely to develop type 2 diabetes. Many other studies point in this direction. In a series of studies involving more than 480,500 individuals followed between 2 and 15 years of age, it is observed that the risk of developing type 2 diabetes is minimal for individuals sleeping between 7 and 8 hours per night[165]. Lack of sleep leads to hormonal cortisol imbalance, which results in long-term harmful hyperglycaemia. Getting enough and quality sleep is essential to reduce the risk of developing diabetes.

Sleep deprivation is a risk factor for cardiovascular disease

People with sleep disorders are at risk of developing high blood pressure. High blood pressure is a disease characterized by excessive pressure in the arteries. High blood pressure is commonly referred to as hypertension for systolic blood pressure (heart contraction) greater than 140 mmHg and diastolic blood pressure (heart relaxation) greater than 90 mmHg. Because of our lifestyle (stress, sedentary lifestyle, diet...), we must pay attention to the risks of contracting high blood pressure. It is important to be informed that if you fail to monitor your blood pressure, especially after age 50, the consequences could lead to a stroke or kidney failure. That's why I usually advise all patients to have blood pressure monitors at home and to learn to use them regularly. There are reliable $60 blood pressure monitors that can measure your heart rate and archive the results daily in your phone.

The time and quality of sleep would have an impact on blood pressure. Studies suggest that people sleeping 5 hours a night, on average, have a greater risk of developing high blood pressure than those sleeping 7 to 8 hours a night. Each hour of sleep lost over five years is associated with a 37% increased risk of high blood pressure[166]. When it becomes customary to shorten sleep because of life's imperatives, there is a high risk of developing high blood pressure in the medium term. Faced with this risk, women are particularly affected. Even mild sleep disorders, such as difficulty falling asleep, can increase blood pressure in women[65] . Artery wall inflammation is also present in the majority of people with very little sleep[166][167]. When sleep disorders last more than 10 years, the risk of developing coronary heart disease is significantly increased[168]. All studies point in the same direction and a genetic predisposition increases the risks in some individuals[169]. Whether it's hypertension, heart disease or stroke: sleep is a key element of our cardiovascular well-being!

Sleep delay is a risk factor for some cancers

This is the case for women working staggered hours, who have warned of the link between cancer and sleep deprivation. Studies of Finnish flight attendants assigned to long-haul flights have shown an increased risk for breast cancer[170]. Data analysis revealed that jet lag was a factor that could explain the 45 breast cancer cases recorded in a sample of more than 1000 women. Then, the studies were extended to other professions working staggered hours such as nurses. Working staggered hours, i.e. night work, leads to a disruption of the internal nycthemeral rhythm, i.e. the body's perception of the succession of day and night. The whole hormonal process is disrupted and in particular the biological rhythm of melatonin, which is secreted between 22:00 and 6:00 in the morning[171]. Transport and health workers working at night are at risk of some cancers. In a study published in 1998, the results showed that 15% of airline flight attendants developed different cancers, with breast cancer cases in the lead[172].

Lack of sleep impacts overall mortality

The lack or alteration of sleep has a very important effect on our general well-being. It is one of the key factors to be controlled in order to avoid triggering the harmful processes that lead to obesity, diabetes, cardiovascular disease and cancer. In developed countries, most deaths are due to heart disease or cancer. During their research, Danish researchers found that adults under 65 years of age who slept less than 5 hours per night had a 65% higher mortality rate than those who slept more than six hours [173]. As soon as you start accumulating sleep debt, the risk of death increases over time. A lack of sleep can double the risk of dying from a heart attack or stroke in people with multiple cardiovascular risk factors such as obesity, hypertension and diabetes. When an individual accumulates cardiovascular risk factors, it is essential to respect the 7 to 9 hours of sleep per night in order to minimize the risk of mortality. Being obese and not getting enough sleep is a risky practice. One solution would be to take advantage of weekends to partially pay off the sleep debts accumulated during the week by practicing catch-up sleep with weekend naps[174].

- ✓ Here are some tips to practice to improve sleep:

- ✓ Meditate regularly even if it is 5 minutes.

- ✓ Move, climb stairs, increase physical activity to generate adenosine and laugh during the day.

- ✓ Last coffee of the day before 2:00.

- ✓ Download filter applications that limit the effects of blue light.

- ✓ Do not use a screen for at least 1 hour before going to bed.

- ✓ Turn off the room screens or at worst disable all sound and vibration signals, relax.

- ✓ Go to bed at regular times.

- ✓ Accept the signs of sleepiness and fatigue (yawning and itchy eyes...), do not resist under the guise of finishing something.

- ✓ Two naps a week, if necessary at weekends for example, to reduce cardiovascular risk and walk in a wooded park or in the forest.
- ✓ A healthy diet.

What are the benefits of sleeping between 7 and 9 hours a night?

Sleep allows for muscle recovery

During a 24-hour day, our body is subjected to a set of cyclical biological events (metabolism, temperature variation, hormone secretion...) called circadian rhythm. Melatonin secreted during sleep is a powerful antioxidant for cell regeneration[175]. An internal clock located in the brain implements a cycle of melatonin secretion under the effect of light[176]. Thanks to melatonin, during the sleep phase, a physical muscular recovery is carried out. The human body has 2 types of muscles: Striated muscles (skeletal and cardiac) and smooth muscles. Good quality sleep is necessary for the recovery of skeletal muscles. Under normal conditions, any degradation of skeletal muscle proteins is compensated by synthesis[177 178]. A circadian cycle deregulation leads to a structural modification of skeletal muscles and consequently to an alteration of muscle performance[179]. A single night of total sleep deprivation is sufficient to trigger a blockage of the genes regulating the muscle body clock[180]. Quality sleep is necessary and essential to activate the genes involved in skeletal muscle repair.

Sleep allows the skin to regenerate itself

More and more scientific studies are showing that sleep allows the skin to regenerate. The role of the skin is to protect us from pollution, ultraviolet rays, and to act as a barrier against anything that can affect our physical integrity. Collagen from the skin plays a major role in this protective function, and its degradation leads to skin ageing[181]. At night and during sleep, the skin regenerates itself because the number of cellular multiplication is at its maximum. During sleep, there is a synthesis of collagen by cells called fibroblasts, with an increase in blood flow to the skin, which results in a radiant complexion in the morning. Sleep deprivation or poor quality sleep accelerates skin aging. Studies have shown that individuals with quality sleep have a higher rate of tissue repair compared to individuals who sleep little[182]. The mechanism is believed to be a dysfunction of immune cells, with the production of chemical and hormonal factors that alter the nocturnal synthesis of collagen[183]. Forty-two hours of sleep deprivation, or a short night, leads to an increase in human cortisol, which inhibits the dermal fibroblasts responsible for collagen synthesis[184]. Over time, the skin will degrade and lose its elasticity and wrinkles can appear in an individual with significant sleep debt. It is important to be aware that it is in the calm of a quality night that the skin regenerates itself.

Sleep limits the production of brain degradation products

Lack of sleep is deleterious to neurons, and can destroy up to 25% of them[185]. Can we deduce from this that an accumulation of sleep debt in humans would have much more serious effects, such as irretrievable alterations in cognitive functions and alertness? Certainly, sleep is necessary for the integrity of the matrix containing the neural networks. Every individual must be aware that from the first night of sleep deprivation, there is a significant accumulation of brain tissue breakdown proteins in the bloodstream. To avoid the buildup of toxic materials in the brain, it is important to maintain good quality sleep, so that the fluid that bathes the brain can fulfill its role as a cleaner[186]. During sleep, the liquid in which the brain is bathed, called cerebrospinal fluid, comes in successive waves to wash and aspirate the toxins from the brain, to send them to the blood that immediately eliminates them. If sleep is of lower quality, this wave cleaning is less effective, with a greater accumulation of toxins[187]. When sleep is impaired, a loss of brain tissue and an accumulation of toxins can explain the long-term onset of neurodegenerative diseases. In view of these elements, it is therefore essential to respect restorative sleep to maintain the tissue integrity of the brain over the long term.

Sleep saves you time to strengthen your knowledge and memory

Sleeping is far from being a loss of time, and the sleep stage is necessary to consolidate knowledge. Thanks to advances in brain imaging, the areas of the brain that are related to learning and that are reactivated during sleep are known. The brain regions active during the awakening phase during a learning process are the same as those that are activated during the sleep that follows this learning process. Learning is "restarted" during the sleep phase, to promote its entry into long-term memory. Consolidation is the process by which newly gained and fragile information is strengthened and/or improved in long-term memory. This consolidation

is due to brain plasticity, i.e. the ability of our brain
to adapt dynamically to integrate new experiences[188].
During daytime learning, the hippocampus, the
structure responsible for long-term memory,
integrates the most important information into a
group of neurons, and eliminates the least important.
Then during sleep, this information is strengthened
and stored in different areas of the cerebral cortex.
Sleep deprivation leads to a deterioration in
information consolidation due to less activation of
the hippocampus. Selective reduction of deep sleep
duration, even without reduction of total sleep
duration, has the same effects[189]. Light sleep (usual in
the elderly), sleep apnea, or simply excessive noise,
are enough to compromise this consolidation of
information. Nevertheless, it has been shown that
short naps, even for less than 1 hour, are sufficient
to consolidate what has just been learned[190]. To
memorize the information as much as possible, it is
enough to remember or relearn the information just
before going to sleep. Consolidation during deep
sleep will produce information integration.

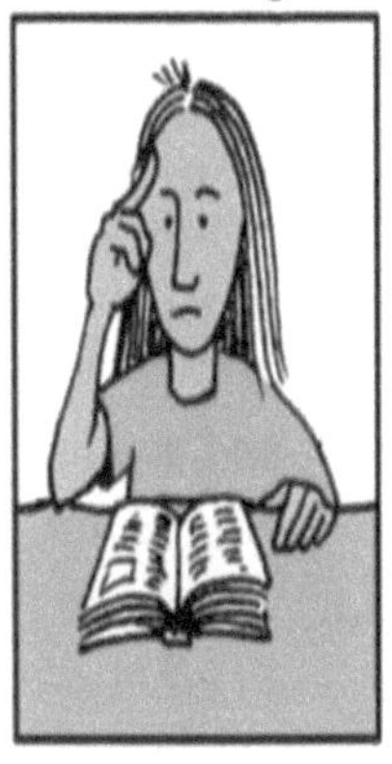

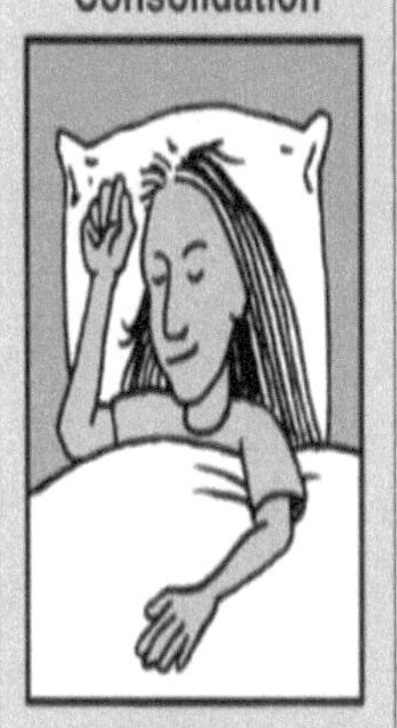

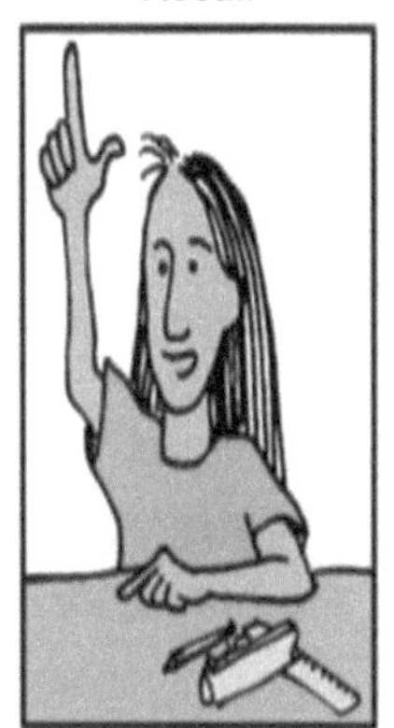

Sleep supports memory consolidation in the brain. The Sleep-Immune Crosstalk in Health and Disease (https://www.physiology.org/doi/full/10.1152/physrev.00010.2018).

Sleep stimulates the immune system

Lack of sleep reduces the immune system and increases the risk of infection. Studies with identical twins confirm this phenomenon, and thus exclude any ideas of genetic predisposition involved

109

in it[191]. For a sleep period of 7 hours, the immune system works optimally. In the event of seasonal epidemics, 7 to 8 hours per night are necessary to recover good health, fairly quickly. If during the winter, you want to avoid as much as possible, all infections during this period, give priority to your sleep.

Lack of sleep promotes inflammatory processes, which are harmful to the body and reduce the immune system. Sleep disorders can lead to the secretion of inflammation triggering factors[192]. These sleep disorders induce an increase in cytokines harmful to the body. These cytokines (usually interleukins 1 and 6 and tumor necrosis factor or TNF Tumor Necrosis Factor) are substances developed by the immune system and are pro-inflammatory, i. e. inflammation triggers[193 194]. Thus, during seasonal flu episodes, this increase in interleukin 6 secretion is particularly observed in individuals suffering from insomnia, against the backdrop of a lack of reactivity of the immune system[195 196]. Fortunately, all hope is not lost. Restoring good nights' sleep allows you to recover the qualities of a good immune system fairly quickly. It is accepted that after 5 successive nights of short duration, a single normal night of 7 to 9 hours will not allow a normal recovery but that it takes more than 3 normal nights for the body to fully recover its performance[197] [198]. If you have poor quality nights, be aware that from the first normal night, your immune system's white blood cells and lymphocytes stabilize quickly[199]. Finally, you can also catch up by taking naps lasting from 30 minutes to 2 hours, which can counteract the effects of some inflammation markers, such as cortisol and interleukin 6[200] [201].

What can I do to get back to quality sleep between 7 and 9 hours a night?

As we have seen, stress and its effects, such as anxiety and depression, are the leading causes of chronic insomnia. Regular physical activity, integrated into lifestyle habits, can help to regain quality sleep. Take action on stress by adopting a physical activity at all times. Even the most minimal activities will have an impact on your sleep. Doing nothing during chronic stress will lead to a gradual increase in cortisol levels in the blood, and install a vicious circle on the brain. Physical activity and meditation can influence decision-making and attention centres. Move and move again, even if in conditions of anxiety and depression, morale does not encourage physical activity. Take the stairs. The practice of group meditation or yoga, are ideal solutions to refocus on oneself in a group dynamic.

Did you know? A molecule, called "adenosine", plays an important role in regulating sleep-wake alternation. When glucose is consumed by the body, it is converted into a substance called adenosine triphosphate (ATP), a real fuel for the body's cells. If a neuron uses this ATP to have energy, adenosine is generated, accumulates in the brain, and will bind to adenosine receptors, causing people to fall asleep.

Be aware of any substance that may affect sleep physiology. The maximum caffeine dose recommendations not to exceed per day for an adult is 400 mg. That is 4 to 5 cups of coffee per day[202.] The caffeine molecule acts on fatigue by displacing the adenosine of its natural receptors in the brain. Thus after 4 to 5 cups of coffee, 50% of the adenosine molecules are moved from their binding site and replaced by caffeine[203]. At this dose of caffeine, no perceptible side effects are noted. For caffeine not to have any effect on sleep quality, it should not be absorbed in the last 6 hours before bedtime[204]. An individual who goes to bed at 10 p.m.

must have his last coffee by 4 p.m. at the latest. Since variations in metabolism are possible between each individual, it is simply better not to take them after 14 hours, in order to guarantee quality sleep. The evening diet should not be too copious. Do not do physical activity late, at the risk of reactivating the metabolism. It is useful to respect fatigue signals when you feel them. The brain gives out signs like yawning, back pain, pushing you to stretch, to signal the need for sleep. Do not oppose it and let yourself be carried away to sleep. Have a temperature between 16 and 22°C in a well ventilated room, calm and switch off all light sources. One of the scourges that disturbs our biological clock is smartphone light. This type of light is a radiation emitted by light-emitting diodes (LEDs) and is found in most digital camera displays. It is known that exposure of the retina to the blue light of the screens deregulates the biological cycle of melatonin. By exposing yourself to the light of digital screens, the natural signs of fatigue will take a long time to express themselves, and will push you to sleep later. Blue light inhibits the initial secretion of melatonin by 55%[205]. However, when darkness sets in, the secretion of melatonin by a small gland located at the back of the brain is necessary to induce sleep. Even if manufacturers recommend using filters, or installing filter applications that partially trap this light in order to limit its impact on sleep, it is essential to turn off these devices at least 1 hour before going to bed[206].

INFLAMMATION

Inflammation is one of the key factors that control the balance of our body. Some people do not mind saying that inflammation is the "mother of all diseases". Most of the disorders of our body are caused by an inflammatory process. Controlling, monitoring and controlling inflammation in a preventive way is the solution to maintain the proper functioning of our cells. Inflammation can wreak havoc on our bodies, and affect our overall health, without us noticing. It is particularly when it becomes chronic that the diseases are most serious. So how can we reduce or avoid this phenomenon, which can cause all kinds of harm and ruin our lives?

Did you know? The inflammatory system is a broad set of physiological reactions, which can occur in almost any tissue of the body. There are 2 types of inflammatory reactions, which are triggered when the body is confronted with bacteria, toxins, injury, or any type of aggression. The first possibility is an acute inflammatory reaction, it is intense and of short duration. When, for example, a bacterial infection occurs, pro-inflammatory molecules activate the immune system, which eliminates the bacteria. Chemical molecules signal the end of the inflammation, and healing is obtained. The second alternative is the chronic inflammatory reaction, it is mild or even asymptomatic and sets in chronically. In this case, low-grade inflammation sets in and despite the presence of immune cells, the body is invaded by an increase in inflammatory reactions, which degenerate into chronic diseases.

So why not simply take anti-inflammatory drugs to prevent or treat these diseases: anti-inflammatory drugs should be taken in high doses, to fight inflammation. For short periods of time, the body tolerates them, which makes it possible to stop inflammation after 7 to 15 days. In the long term, they are toxic to the digestive tract, causing, for example, very serious ulcers or serious heart problems such as myocardial infarction. Finally, some drugs, such as corticosteroids, can cause very serious metabolic disorders. This is why the prescription of these drugs is limited in time, or must be extremely monitored, if they are prescribed over the long term.

Chronic inflammation leads to neurodegenerative diseases

Neurodegenerative diseases are distinguished by a deterioration in the functioning of nerve cells, particularly neurons. One of the most well-known diseases is Alzheimer's disease. If you could look at the brain of a person with Alzheimer's disease, you would see that some areas are atrophied. This results in a loss of memory, ability to think, as well as strange and inconsistent behaviour. It affected about 26 million people worldwide in 2005, and could reach four times as many in 2050[207]. More and more studies are linking permanent inflammation with neurodegenerative diseases. Researchers find that the decline in brain function is generally related to an accumulation of inflammation proteins[208] [209]. High levels of interleukin 6, for example, are very closely related to the decline in brain function observed in a population followed for 10 years[208]. As early as the age of 50, the decline in brain performance begins[210]. Beyond age 55, high levels of an inflammation marker, the C-reactive protein, follow cognitive decline[210]. The possibility that a person will trigger Alzheimer's disease 20 to 30 years later can be predicted with some certainty, as this chronicity of inflammation most often leads to this type of dementia[211]. The coincidence between these early markers of inflammation, and the amyloid plaques observed in Alzheimer's disease, suggests a very strong link between inflammation and neurodegenerative diseases[212].

Chronic inflammation contributes to type 2 diabetes

Diabetes is a chronic disease caused by a lack of, or failure to use insulin. Recent studies have shown that it is a chronic inflammatory phenomenon, which is the cause of type 2[213] diabetes. While the risk factors (obesity, lack of physical activity, foods high in saturated fats, etc.) are almost everyone's responsibility, many people are unaware that this is a low-grade inflammatory phenomenon that takes root in chronicity. In addition, obese and diabetic people very often have certain types of immune cells involved in inflammation in their circulating blood. These immune cells are also implicated in the modification of the intestinal flora of obese and diabetic patients[214]. The control of the cellular and hormonal elements involved in chronic inflammation is a solution to prevent diabetes.

Chronic inflammation results in cardiovascular disease

Chronic and intrusively evolving inflammation is also involved in cardiovascular disease[215]. Since the 1970s, a very strong link has been established between excess cholesterol in the blood and the formation of atheroma plaques[216]. The deposition of these plaques in the arteries induces a phenomenon called atherosclerosis. It leads to serious diseases such as myocardial infarction and stroke. The strategy for the management of these diseases is to reduce bad cholesterol, in order to reduce the risk of these cardiovascular diseases. But unfortunately, the real impact of lowering this bad cholesterol on these diseases is minor[217 218]. The only hypothesis of excess cholesterol, in the understanding of cardiovascular disease, has shown limitations. Studies have focused on the involvement of chronic inflammatory phenomena, as markers of chronic inflammation are almost present in patients affected by these cardiovascular diseases, and in the development of atheroma plaque. Patients who have undergone well-conducted treatments with statin, a drug known to be effective on cholesterol, often end up with residual markers of inflammation that are harmful to cardiovascular health[219]. As we have seen for diabetes, beyond risk factors such as obesity, physical inactivity and diet, consideration of chronic inflammation is necessary to adopt the right preventive strategies against cardiovascular disease.

Chronic inflammation results in osteoarticular diseases

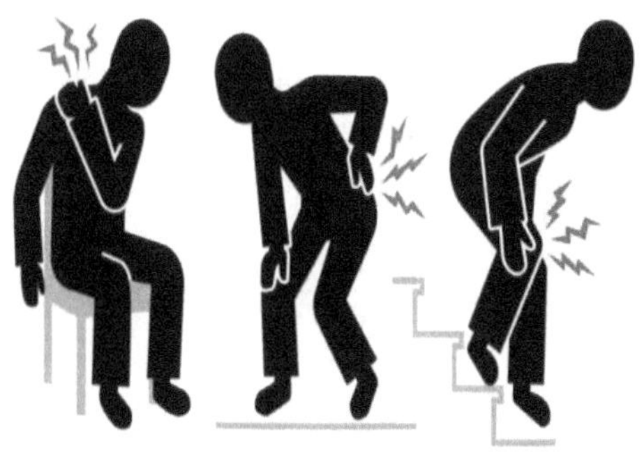

Some osteoarticular pathologies are distinguished by the presence of signs of inflammation. These pathologies are diverse and the most well-known are rheumatoid arthritis, osteoarthritis and osteoporosis... Until 2016, these pathologies were the second most important and disabling diseases after mental illnesses[220]. What characterizes them is the presence of pain. These diseases can affect young people. The triggers for these diseases are weight, physical inactivity, genetics or stress. Globally, 10 to 15% of the population is affected. In 2018, nearly 37% of American adults under 65 years of age are affected by osteoarthritis[221]. These diseases have an impact on quality of life, sleep, but also mortality due to the sedentary lifestyle they cause. In osteoarthritis, for example, at the joints, the surface of the cartilage cracks, crumbles and eventually disappears. An insidious and chronic inflammation will gradually develop and prevent the physiological reconstruction of cartilage cells. The joint is attacked by pro-inflammatory cytokines, interleukin-1 and TNF-α[222]. The statistics are alarming and the disease is seriously disabling. By 2040, 25% of Americans will be reached[223]. Il est nécessaire d'adopter un mode de vie permettant de prévenir l'émergence de ces pathologies ostéo-articulaires.

Chronic inflammation leads to intestinal pathologies

Chronic inflammation can also affect the digestive tract. It will manifest itself in most cases in the form of 2 diseases: Crohn's disease and hemorrhagic rectocolitis. These diseases are mainly found in the countries of the northern hemisphere, and the number of new cases is increasing[224]. About 3 million Americans and 2 million Europeans are currently affected by these diseases, and the emergence of new cases is due to industrialization, and to a caloric diet containing saturated fatty acids and low fibre[225]. In the United States, the discovery of these diseases in the majority of individuals occurs between the ages of 20 and 39, with a second peak around the age of 60[226]. All risk factors, i.e. the environment, stress, genetic dispositions, the immune system and infectious agents, have an effect on the microbial intestinal flora[227]. Individuals who consume caloric foods, high in saturated fatty acids and low in fibre, are at greater risk of developing these intestinal diseases[228]. This type of extremely caloric diet triggers inflammatory processes by modifying the intestinal flora, with high concentrations of cytokines typical of inflammation[229] [230] [231].

The consideration of the microbial flora and the control of the food, are decisive elements for the control of the inflammatory process.

Chronic inflammation results in respiratory diseases

Chronic respiratory diseases can impact lung structures. Hundreds of millions of people suffer from chronic respiratory diseases every day. According to WHO estimates, 235 million people currently have asthma, 64 million have chronic obstructive pulmonary disease (COPD), i.e. irreversible narrowing of the bronchi, while millions more suffer from allergic rhinitis, and other chronic respiratory diseases that are often undiagnosed. The factors favouring these pathologies are often environmental factors, with pollution and tobacco in the forefront. These pollutants induce a chronic low-grade inflammation, which over the years will lead to serious diseases. In a smoker, the contact of tobacco components with the bronchi and alveoli, which they attack, activates the recruitment of inflammatory and immune cells from the lung[232]. The long-term consequences are extremely harmful to the health of individual smokers. Frequent exposure to these contaminants will lead to slow and progressive obstruction of the airways and lungs with harmful changes in the alveoli[233]. Worse still, the consequences of these pulmonary changes can lead to sudden death in adults[234]. In the case of asthma, the evolution towards chronicity and aggravation is generally characterized by the presence of inflammatory cells but also by the release of associated mediators who are responsible for inflammation of the respiratory tract, and its consequences. What is also unique about asthma is the presence of eosinophilic cells during episodes of worsening asthma. In adults, an increase in the number of eosinophils in sputum has been observed during aggravations of the disease[235 236]. Recruitment of these eosinophils is controlled by pro-inflammatory cytokines[237]. Chronic exposure to environmental pollutants is a major issue in health prevention. It can cancel out all the efforts made by any individual to maintain good health: even through regular physical activity, any individual constantly exposed to tobacco smoke or other pollutants increases his risk of respiratory diseases. Direct exposure of lung cells to pollutants has a major impact on life expectancy. The most effective prevention strategy must first avoid exposure of lung tissue to inflammation stimulants.

Chronic inflammation is involved in most cancers

Carcinogenesis is the set of phenomena that transform a normal cell into a cancerous cell. It is a long multi-step process, involving changes in the DNA of healthy cells, and can take more than 10 years to manifest as diseases[238]. Some products to which we are exposed on a daily basis can be transformed by enzymes in the body, and cause toxic action on the genome. The transformation of these products leads to the formation of reactive derivatives that will be grafted onto the genome[239]. These are chemical compounds called polycyclic aromatic hydrocarbons (PAHs), which are produced mainly by tobacco smoke and vehicle exhaust gases. Grilling meat at high temperatures leads to the formation of these reactive products[240]. Repeated exposure of our body to these products will generally lead to skin, lung, urinary and digestive tract cancers.

Apart from these toxic substances, another phenomenon occurs spontaneously in our cells. This

126

is oxidative stress, the excess of which causes cancer. Oxidative stress occurs mainly in our mitochondria, and its deleterious nature is linked to the excessive production of reactive oxygen and nitrogen derivatives. These reactive derivatives stimulate the production of 2 cytoplasmic factors Nrf2/Keap1 which control the transformation of healthy cells into cancer cells.

Did you know? Nrf2 (Nuclear factor erythroid-derived 2) located in the cell cytoplasm has the ability to enter the cell nucleus, and to activate or inhibit genes that regulate oxidative stress. Activation of Nrf2 factor can regulate more than 600 genes, including more than 200 coding for proteins, with a protective effect in various diseases, such as cancer and neurodegenerative diseases.

Keap1 (Kelch-like ECH-associated protein1) binds to Nrf2 protein to neutralize it in the cellular cytoplasm[241]. These 2 factors are the subject of intense research for the discovery of drugs that can act on oxidative stress.

The chronic inflammatory phenomenon stimulates immune cells, such as macrophages, eosinophils, lymphocytes, etc. It is estimated that 25% of cancer cases are related to a process involving chronic infection or inflammation[242]. It is a necessary response to deal with aggression. The response involves different immune cells, and preponderant cytokines such as TNF, interleukins 1 and 6 in the first instance, to maintain tissue integrity. Thus, in the face of any aggression of our tissues, the secretion of these factors leads to the migration of the body's defence cells, which come to perform a cleaning role for the aggressor agent. Once the attacking agent is removed, other factors are secreted, so that the defence cells stop the elimination process. However, inappropriate responses may occur, or an excess of cytokines evolving at low noise may occur and become chronic. Most of the time, it is because of repeated infections, obesity, exposure to major pollutants or even the presence of a deleterious gene. Chronic inflammation leads to DNA damage. During the active phase of several cancers (breast, myeloma, prostate...), the secretion of pro-inflammatory cytokines is accompanied by the presence of proteins called NF-kB factors[243]. These factors activate DNA into RNA, for the synthesis of proteins that support the proliferation of cancer cells[244]. Other pro-inflammatory factors, mainly located in the nuclei of the cancer cell, and having identical roles to those of NF-kB factors are also involved. These are, for example, the factors PPARγ involved in lipid metabolism[245]. When it comes to preventing cancer, it is essential to avoid the development of chronic inflammation at all costs. An anti-inflammatory lifestyle is at the heart of prevention.

How can chronic inflammation be reversed very quickly?

Limit sugars and harmful fatty acids

One of the first steps to reverse chronic inflammation is to ban certain foods. These foods induce the production of pro-inflammatory cytokines and intensify oxidative stress. All these processes lead to an excessive formation of NF-kB[246]. The production of all these pro-inflammatory factors is found during the acute phase of many diseases[247]. In most obese people, oxidative stress is particularly important, especially when the diet is high in calories with an excessive intake of fast sugars and saturated and trans fatty acids[248] [249] [250].

Sugars provide us with most of the energy we need. To reverse chronic inflammation, the diet should include sugars that do not suddenly raise blood sugar levels. It has been noted that the diet based on refined rice, which has a high glycemic index, induces significant oxidative stress with, as a consequence, a high rate of diabetes in Asian populations[251] [252] [253]. The researchers found that sudden changes in blood glucose levels stimulate chronic inflammation and oxidative stress in adipocytes[254] [255]. Similarly, epidemiological studies[256] [257] have confirmed the link between caloric, high sugar diet and chronic inflammatory conditions such as diabetes and obesity. That's why if you want to stop the inflammation that is smouldering in your body, the first simple step is to keep so-called fast sugars out of the diet. These fast sugars are mainly found in foods that give you an immediate taste of sweet sodas, industrial cakes, spreads and sweets. They are also hidden in some foods such as industrial recipes and chocolate bars for example. Sugars will be brought to the body through the consumption of whole grains that avoid sudden changes in blood sugar levels. These include, for example, spelt and oatmeal flakes, whole wheat, whole grain rice, quinoa, etc... Whole grains have a fibrous envelope that has a beneficial effect by reducing calories absorbed, weight, and risk of type 2 diabetes by 23%[258] [259].

For harmful fatty acids, the first control point is to avoid as much as possible processed foods containing trans fats. These trans fatty acids are true oxidative stress bombs[260]. Our body has absolutely no need for them. Their use in industrial food has led to an explosion in cardiovascular diseases[261].

These trans fats occur naturally in fats, ruminant meats and dairy products such as butter, yogurt and milk. That is why the consumption of meat and dairy products should not be excessive. But the worst is the trans fatty acids manufactured by the agri-food industry to stabilize and preserve food over the long term. Although regulations restricting their use exist in most countries, such as Canada, the United States and various European countries, it is important to limit the consumption of industrial products in order not to quickly reach significant amounts in the blood[262]. WHO recommends that total trans fat intakes should not exceed 1% of total energy intakes, or less than 2.2 gr/day for a 2000 calorie diet[263].

They are found in several products: breads, sandwiches, breakfast cereals, cakes, industrial soups, frozen dishes... But also in all types of preparations involving processing techniques, such as frying or grilling. Oils should not be heated to excessive temperatures over long periods of time at the risk of generating trans fatty acids. A high consumption of red or processed meats also generates toxic compounds, especially when these meats are grilled[264]. This phenomenon is often blamed for the occurrence of colorectal cancers[265]. Just the daily consumption of 50 g of red meat increases the risk of cancer by 18%[247].

Saturated fatty acids also stimulate oxidative stress[266] [267] [268]. A diet high in saturated fat induces a disruption of mitochondria in many organs, with the production of intense oxidative stress[269] [270] [271]. Most of our cells need fatty acids to form their membrane, and our needs are estimated at 30 g per day. The consumption of a single croissant provides 15 grams of saturated fat, half of your daily requirement. Unfortunately, any excess of red meat, butter, cold cuts, dairy products, lard... leads to direct fatty acid deposits in the arteries... Over time, these deposits will lead to atheroma plaques, with local stimulation of inflammatory phenomena, whose consequences are catastrophic for the heart and brain. It is important to moderate the consumption of foods containing excess saturated fatty acids. Butter, for example, is very rich in saturated fatty acids: in 100 g of butter, there are more than 60 g of saturated fats, and it is especially important to avoid heating it so as not to generate even more trans fatty acids. Favouring good fats, and lowering sources of saturated and trans fatty acids are necessary conditions to limit chronic inflammation. For that, olive oil must simply be the bottle of oil you need to have in your kitchen, at any time. It is rich in monounsaturated fatty acids, vitamin E and other antioxidants that give it anti-inflammatory properties with a real impact on the heart and vessels, especially when it comes to extra virgin olive oil[272]. Olive oil can be used for frying, provided that the temperature is not increased too much. The temperatures not to be exceeded are indicated on the labels: in general 238°C for ordinary olive oil and 191°C for extra virgin olive oil. By exceeding these temperatures, fatty acids are degraded and generate toxic compounds. To keep intact during frying, vitamin E and most antioxidants, it is recommended not to exceed 180°C, which is usually the average frying temperature[273].

You must pay attention to the quality of olive oil, by reading the labels carefully, because adulterated, lower quality products are circulating on the market.

For breakfast in the morning: wholemeal bread in olive oil

It is essential to moderate butter consumption. For breakfast, it is possible to alternate with wholemeal bread in extra virgin olive oil. To do this, take a few slices of wholemeal bread and simply spread with a few drops of olive oil. You can add nuts to enhance the taste. I do not recommend toasting wholemeal bread to avoid any formation of acrylamide, a product that increases the risk of cancer.

Currently, some margarines benefit from better manufacturing technology, which limits the trans acid content to less than 1%, and without palm oil. These margarines enriched in polyunsaturated acids, omega-3, can also be alternated with butter and wholemeal bread in olive oil.

Maintain the balance of the intestinal flora with omega-3 fatty acids

The intestinal flora is very concerned with inflammatory phenomena[227]. We talked about how it influences the weight of individuals. Other specialists go beyond that, and see it as the body's "second brain". Composed mainly of billions of bacteria that live in symbiosis in the body, this intestinal flora plays a major role in controlling inflammation and the immune system. It has been shown that when the intestinal mucosa loses its bacteria, its intestinal immune function collapses[274]. Worse still, the effect may be on the whole body with a collapse of lymphocytic cells, which circulate in the general circulation[275]. Bacteria in the intestinal flora play a role in the genesis of inflammation. This role can be beneficial as deleterious, depending on the conditions to which they are regularly subjected. It has been shown that the bacteria *Faecalibacterium prausnitzii,* for example, is a good bacterium of the digestive tract and is believed to play a protective role in Crohn's disease[276]. An imbalance between intestinal tissues and bacterial flora can increase the risk of diseases such as diabetes, chronic intestinal diseases, colorectal cancers and neurodegenerative pathologies of the Alzheimer type[277] [278] [279]. More and more evidence shows that it is our diet that regulates the quality of the intestinal flora. There are two types of polyunsaturated fatty acids that our bodies cannot produce: Omega-3 and Omega-6 fatty acids. The diet must provide them with an omega3/omega-6 ratio of about 1/5 maximum in order to avoid harmful consequences for the body[280]. Individuals with normal levels of omega-3 have a balanced flora, and are less prone to chronic inflammatory diseases[281]. Omega-3 fatty acids are found in large quantities in certain fatty fish such as salmon, sardines, chia seeds and flax, walnuts, camelina and rapeseed... As for omega-6, they are mainly of vegetable origin, and the quantity necessary for the proper functioning of the body is low.

Modern diets are low in omega-3, and are distinguished by ratios in the order of 1/10 or 1/20[282] [283]. It is therefore essential to consume foods that provide omega-3 intakes, in order to restore the normal ratio of 1/5, because these acids have anti-inflammatory properties[284]. The daily requirement of omega-3 for an adult is 1.3 grams per day, which corresponds to one tablespoon (15 ml) of rapeseed oil or 100 grams of fatty fish per week. To achieve the right omega-3/omega-6 ratio, it is sufficient to consume 1 portion of 25 g of nuts (1 portion = 5 to 8 kernels or a handful) per day, and to also have rapeseed oil for seasoning. Be careful, this oil does not tolerate temperatures above 150°C. Omega-3-based dietary supplements do not have a direct beneficial effect on cardiovascular problems[285]. Worse still, most consumers are unaware that the omega-3s contained in the capsules can be quickly degraded[286] and that whole natural products should be preferred. The balance of the intestinal flora being an essential condition for good health, it must be maintained by a regular supply of omega-3, in order to slow down the secretion of pro-inflammatory factors.

Diet rich in various fruits and vegetables providing at least 30 g of fibre and 500 mg of flavonoids per day

The consumption of fibre and vegetables helps to reduce the effects of stress, and to fight chronic inflammation. People who regularly consume these products are at lower risk of cardiovascular disease and cancer. Concerning fibres, we have expanded their impact on the composition of the intestinal flora. The beneficial effects require daily quantities of about 30 g per day, because it is from this quantity that the bacterial flora is qualitatively modified. As a reminder, the Western diet provides an average of 15 grams of fibre per day. Another important indicator is that the power supply must be coloured! Red, green, yellow... since fruit and vegetables are part of the diet, it must be varied in colour or at least alternated regularly. These colours are due to pigments, the most important of which are flavonoids and carotenoids. They are found in pumpkins, carrots, peppers, tomatoes, onions, broccoli, green tea, parsley, celery, citrus fruits, apples, red fruits, soybeans...and even in dark chocolate[287].

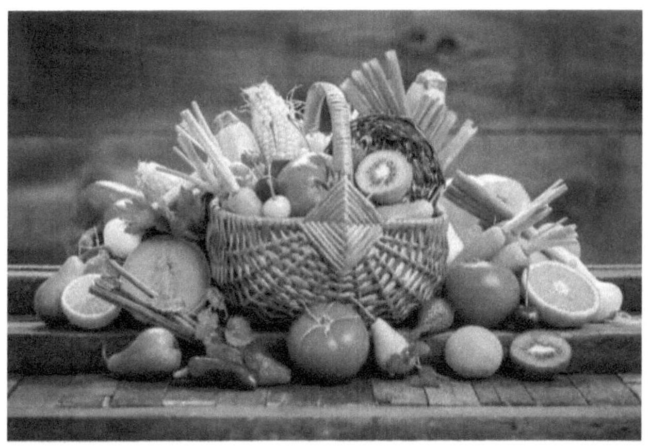

The flavonoids contained in fruits and vegetables have a major role in the fight against chronic inflammation. They exert their anti-inflammatory action by inhibiting the entire cascade of reactions leading to the activation of NF-kB factors[288]. Action on other transcription factors involved in chronic inflammation is also reported[289]. Follow-up studies in patients with colorectal cancer have shown that consumption of more than 30 mg of flavonoids per day reduces cytokines that mark inflammation[290 291]. While the effect on inflammation markers is significant, a Danish study shows that it is from 500 mg of consumption per day that flavonoids have a significant impact on the risk of

mortality from cancer and cardiovascular disease[287].
To reach the 500 mg flavonoid target, a daily intake
of either one apple, one orange, one portion of
broccoli, one portion of berries or two cups of green
tea is sufficient. Variability of fruits and vegetables
must be the rule.

The principle of an anti-inflammatory diet

It is important to eat fresh produce (fruit, vegetables,
meat, fish, eggs, etc.)

Sweets, chocolate bars, pastries, crisps, ready-made
or frozen meals, ice creams, sweetened drinks induce
inflammation factors[257].

BREAKFAST

Replace fruit juice with a fruit mixture. Eat whole
fruits to benefit from their fibre. Crush the banana:
Crushing the banana will oxidize it. Banana is one of
the few fruits that becomes even better with
oxidation.

Make mixtures of 3 to 5 fruits cut into small pieces
(1 Apple, 1 Banana, 5 blueberries for example) with
a small quantity of rapeseed oil.

Add nuts (a few squash seeds, chia seeds, cashews for example: for iron, calcium, and unsaturated fatty acids that protect the cardiovascular system). Wholemeal bread can be spread with extra virgin olive oil.

Around 10:00 am (optional)

Almonds or dark chocolate (80% cocoa) to snack on in the middle of the morning or dried fruit! An apple of organic origin is a good idea!

LUNCH AND DINNER (Drink at least 2 x 125 ml glasses of water before and during meals; the last coffee of the day must be taken before 2 p.m)

A meal must be composed of 5 types of food: whole grains, animal protein, legumes, virgin oil, vegetables.
– Whole grains: Choice of quinoa, pasta, rice, millet, semolina, bread, buckwheat,... Why whole grains?
Low glycemic index, richer in vitamins and minerals. For bread, prefer wholemeal bread, cereal bread, rye, buckwheat or spelt bread.
– 1 protein preferably based on fish: only one per meal. Why a protein? 20% reduction in the risk of stroke by providing vitamin B1[237],
- 1 legume: beans, lentils...
- 1 virgin oil (cold pressed): olive oil for example

- 1 MINIMUM vegetable. The ideal way is to start your meal with a raw vegetable (salads, for example). A small salad of raw vegetables as a starter with cider vinegar, walnut oil or olive oil and turmeric powder, then the main course with steamed vegetables, steaming preserving the nutrients of the vegetable best.

Chewing well: Chewing is good health.

Others: Learn to avoid salt (the diet already contains enough salt), and do not accompany with alcohol

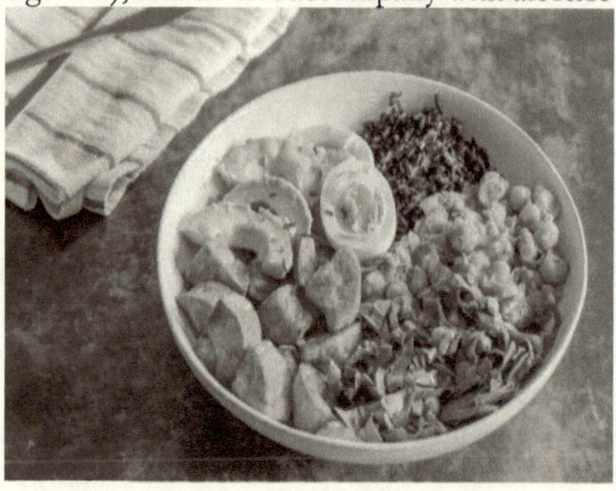

Maintain regular physical activity

Fighting chronic inflammation also means maintaining regular physical activity. Moderate physical activity reduces the markers of chronic inflammation. A clear distinction must be made here between acute and chronic stress. As we have mentioned, chronic stress is an undetectable process, which takes place over long periods of time while causing deleterious effects, which will lead to chronic diseases much later. Physical activity reduces the effects of reactive compounds, helping the immune system to eliminate them. Involvement in physical activities is a potential risk of musculoskeletal injuries. They are often perceived as a source of stress. But, it must be taken into account that moderate and progressive physical activity is excellent, to cancel the harmful effects of chronic stress even if the results are not immediately visible. After a short moderate exercise of 20 minutes, you decrease the production of the pro-inflammatory TNFα by 5%[292]. A 20-minute brisk walk produces this effect. These 20 minutes are the minimum time required to trigger at least 5% anti-inflammatory activity. If you want to have more impact, you have to do more in terms of time, until you reach 1 hour of moderate activity. The longer you increase the duration of moderate exercise, the more there is a decrease in the production of pro-inflammatory TNFα[293]. This is why you should not hesitate to take the 7500 steps per day, between 30 and 60 minutes, in order to benefit from a maximum daily anti-inflammatory effect.

How can we prevent or better live with lung cancer?

It is when we manage the treatment of lung cancer patients that we become aware of the damage caused by tobacco. While at the end of my internship at the hospital, I did a year of training in pulmonology, I had to follow chemotherapy courses for patients with lung cancer, in order to ensure the proper preparation of drugs for the next courses of treatment. I have only one thing to say: run away from tobacco! Or make the necessary efforts to get out. The figures are clear: lung cancers in 90% of cases, in developed countries, tobacco is the cause[294]. It is also the most deadly cancer in the world. Each year, there are 1.35 million new cases detected, and 1.18 million deaths, with the highest rates in Europe and North America. In the prevention strategy, quitting smoking is crucial. Physical activity can help people cope with the disease by reducing symptoms such as fatigue. The most active patients also see their quality of life improve through improved physical fitness[295]. A patient with lung cancer, or even narrowing of the bronchi due to smoking, can improve his or her respiratory capacity after 4 weeks of regular physical activity, which allows him or her to be in better conditions to cope with the disease[296] [297]. Since patients' respiratory capacity is reduced by the disease, regular and moderate walking of 30 to 60 minutes per day is sufficient to improve patients' quality of life[298] [299]. Even among patients diagnosed at an early stage of the disease, who have received chemotherapy for 5 years, those who have received regular physical exercise are significantly less affected by fatigue and anxiety[300]. Certainly, physical exercise in patients with lung cancer stimulates the immune system, and leads to the evacuation of pro-inflammatory factors[301].

Diet has a considerable role in the prevention of lung cancer. But quitting smoking remains essential. A varied and daily diet of more than 5 fruits and vegetables is associated with a 23% lower risk of lung cancer[302]. A synthesis of studies concludes that risk reductions are around 14% among smokers, when fruit and vegetable consumption is around 400 g per day[303]. But it is not because we have good eating habits, and we regularly exercise, that we can allow ourselves to smoke. It is important to specify for smokers that attention should be paid to beta-carotene, which is found in high doses in food supplements, to facilitate skin tanning. Beta-carotene is converted into vitamin A once ingested and the daily requirement is 2 mg. It has an important role in night vision. It is also involved in a wide range of body functions, such as growth, tissue renewal (skin, intestinal mucosa), or the immune system, in wound healing processes, and protects the skin from external aggressions, such as the sun. Among smokers, long-term consumption of dietary supplements containing non-nutritional doses of beta-carotene (20 to 30 mg/d) significantly increases the risk of lung cancer[304].

How can metastases in breast cancer be prevented or delayed as much as possible?

Breast cancer is the most common cancer found in women[305]. The risk increases significantly with age, between 30 and 60 years of age. 5 to 10% of these cancers have a hereditary genetic origin; 85% to 90% of cases have environmental or unknown origins. Among the non-genetic causes identified were the use of certain estrogen and progesterone drugs, a diet high in sugars, saturated fatty acids, obesity, alcohol consumption and lack of physical activity. Prevention is essential. When properly conducted, it helps to avoid the disease, or to treat it when it is at an early stage. For example, few women know that alcohol raises the risk of breast cancer[306]. Similarly, women should be encouraged to engage in physical activity, and to avoid working staggered hours.[170] Indeed, engaging in physical activity for 30 to 60 minutes a day reduces the risk of breast cancer by 30 to 40%[307]. And what is still interesting is that the more intense the physical activities, the more the risk reduction increases. Thus, more than 5 hours of intense activity reduces the risk by more than 38%, even for women with a family history or those who have not had children[308]. The link between breast cancer and physical activity is through weight regulation, and more specifically fat mass control. Indeed, the excess of intra-abdominal fat increases estrogen production tenfold, by an enzyme called aromatase. This excess of estrogen, for long periods of time, transforms breast cells into cancer cells. Intense sporting activity leads to a significant decrease in estrogen production[309]. For patients already suffering from the disease and benefiting from chemotherapy, physical exercise makes it possible to improve quality of life and better cope with care by reducing anxiety[310 311]. As we have pointed out for alcohol, as a risk factor, quitting smoking is also necessary[312]. It is important to avoid fast sugars and saturated fats from the diet, in other words, industrial food. To this end, the contribution of fruit and vegetables must be the priority. A woman who consumes more than 5 servings of fruits and vegetables per day, or more than 400 grams, reduces the risk of breast cancer by 11%, compared to a woman who consumes half as much. This reduction in cancer risk also concerns aggressive tumours, those with statuses called "ER-negative tumours" for Estrogen Receptor negative, i. e. without estrogen receptors, and positive for HER2[313] receptors. These are cruciferous vegetables such as broccoli, yellow vegetables and oranges, that are most associated with a reduced risk of breast cancer. The antioxidants contained in these fruits and vegetables play a key role in reducing risk. Concerning weight, any variation in the direction of a decrease or an increase is a factor of poor prognosis. The diet should stabilize the weight[314]. Special attention should be paid when breast cancer is classified as "triple negative" (no estrogen, progesterone and epidermal growth factor receptors). These cancers are situations, where there are no known markers on the surface of breast cancer cells that can respond to a known targeted therapy. In other words, it is like a cancer that would only respond to hard chemotherapy, and where there are few places for immunotherapy. In this case, it is important that the patient avoid certain foods that accelerate the progression of the disease. Patients with breast cancer should limit asparagine intake to reduce the spread of the disease. But this amino acid is present in a large part of our diet, and such a diet is difficult to follow. Foods rich in asparagine should be avoided, as this amino acid seems to accelerate the formation of metastases, which enter the bloodstream to colonize the lungs, brain or liver[315]. Patients with breast cancer, especially triple negative breast cancer, should have a preference for fresh fruits and vegetables, corn, rice and wholemeal bread. Asparagus, industrial products dried by heat and fan must be discarded, as they contain a high content of asparagine. The choice must be for foods containing less than 450 picomoles of asparagine/mg of food.

Name of the product	Picomole/ mg
Heat-dried apricots	35000
Heat-dried asparagus	18000
Heat-dried apple	11000
Heat-dried banana	4000
Fan-dried apricots	3000
Fan-dried asparagus	2500
Raw red potatoes	790
Fan-dried apple	**425**
Boiled red potatoes	**200**
Raw potatoes	**170**
Boiled potatoes	150
Raw fishing	**60**
Raw blueberry	**50**
Raw apple	**40**
Raw maize	**20**
Inside of the bread	**18**
Boiled rice	**10**
Boiled corn	**10**
Bread crust	**5**

Asparagine level per mg of food (for breast cancer, prefer foods containing less than 450 picomoles of asparagine/mg of food).

How to prevent or better live with prostate cancer?

Prostate cancer is less prevalent in South Asia and the Far East, and more prevalent in Europe and the United States. According to the American Cancer Society, this cancer is rarer in Asians, and more common in black people. Prostate cancer most often occurs after the age of 50. Overall, it is the second most common cancer in humans[316]. In addition to genetic factors, other factors such as testosterone levels, milk, butter, excessive calcium intake, physical activity, sleep and smoking are mentioned. In the first studies, the impact of physical activity on reducing prostate cancer risk was estimated to be between 10% and 30%[317] [318]. It was recognized that only fairly vigorous and regular physical activity could have a protective role in prostate cancer. With hindsight and years of observation, physical activity seems to be rather beneficial in patients with the disease, with the beneficial effect of reducing the risk of progression and mortality. The risk of mortality is reduced by 30% to 40% compared to men who were not active. We could see that those who were active had a better survival[319]. For this reason, for men about 70 years old, 30 to 60 minutes a day of moderate activity, such as cycling or walking, is necessary.

Food is important in prevention. Regular consumption of dairy products rich in calcium should be avoided in adult men from the age of 50[320]. Alcohol consumption should be reduced and remain exceptional. As for tobacco, it must simply be eliminated, as it is involved in most aggressive cancers. A diet containing portions of mushrooms twice a week, starting at age 50, reduces the risk of prostate cancer by 8%, regardless of their consumption of fruits and vegetables, meat and dairy products15. This risk is reduced by 17% if consumption is reduced to three times a week. This effect is due to the beneficial and antioxidant action of L-ergothionein. This means incorporating about 80 g of fresh mushrooms (button mushrooms, Shiitake, Maitake, Enoki...) into the fruit and vegetables three times a week. The consumption of fatty acids with anti-inflammatory properties, derived from fatty fish such as farmed salmon, should be avoided, as these farms are likely to contain toxic pollutants involved in prostate cancer[321]. If the origin of the fish is not controlled, the simplest choice is to prefer products of vegetable origin, i.e. olive oil, rapeseed oil or walnuts.

How to prevent or better live colorectal cancer?

Gastrointestinal cancers include esophageal, stomach, liver, gastrointestinal stroma and colorectal cancers. It is now accepted that the majority of these cancers are linked to chronic infectious and inflammatory processes[322]. These cancers are on the rise worldwide, with a higher rate of new cases for colorectal cancers (the third most common cancer in the world) and pancreatic cancer[305]. In developed countries, 90% of stomach cancer cases are linked to the proliferation of the bacteria *Helicibacter pylori*[323]. Physical activity has also been shown to be effective in colon cancer. Occasionally, growths, called polyps, form on the mucous membrane of the colon. These growths can develop into colon cancer. One hour of physical activity per week reduces the risk of colon cancer due to degeneration of intestinal polyps[324]. During physical activity, it is an activation of the cells of the immune system, which would allow a reduction of colon polyps[325]. In a synthesis of analyses, it is shown that individuals who are active 7 hours a day have a reduced risk of 24% of colon cancer[326]. Beyond 7 hours of activity per day, the risks are even lower, reaching 40%[327]. There is insufficient data to conclude for rectal cancer[328]. Diet can play a very important role in cancer risk, especially for colorectal cancer. As mentioned above, limited consumption of red meat and processed meat is necessary to reduce the risk of colorectal cancer. It is important to limit alcohol consumption, avoid smoking and control weight. Calcium intake should be limited to what is strictly necessary to reduce the risk of colorectal cancer. Calcium is an essential mineral for maintaining bone health and regulating blood pressure. The results of some cancer studies suggest that low calcium intake increases the risk of colorectal cancer[329]. Calcium intake in adults should be about 900 mg per day and can be provided by vegetables, fruits, or seafood. But beware, calcium intake through dairy products is not recommended especially for men over 50 years of age, because of the risks of prostate cancer[320]. For this reason, a diet based on fruits and vegetables is an excellent alternative, especially since they also provide fibre.

List of some vegetables, fruits, or seafood products to add to your recipes to ensure an adequate calcium intake.

Seafood products as a source of calcium for 100 g of products

Sardine in oil 798 mg

Salmon 270 mg

Shrimp 240 mg

Scallop 220 mg

Anchovies 189 mg

Flat oyster 186 mg

Calcium source vegetables per 100 g of vegetables

Leeks 252 mg

Curly kale 185 mg

Spinach 159 mg

Rocket 129 mg

Cress 110 mg

White bean 183 mg

Beans 103 mg

Fruits and seeds as sources of calcium per 100 g of fruit

Almond 266 mg

Brazil nuts 150 mg

Hazelnut 123 mg

Chia 631 mg

Fibre intake is particularly well known against colon cancer. The effect is so dramatic that when a person consuming enough fibre adopts a low-fibre diet, the markers of inflammation appear after 15 days[330]! The Western diet provides, on average, only 15 grams of fibre per day, while the daily intake should be about 30 grams. As we have said, to lose weight, it is important to eat the whole fruit and vegetables, to ensure fibre intake. Beyond the preventive effect, an individual with colon cancer can reduce the risk of early death by 22% by increasing his daily fibre intake by 5gr[331]. And we must take advantage of this to ensure an adequate supply of flavonoids, through coloured fruits and vegetables, which are antioxidants and anti-inflammatory! Vegetables providing 400 mg of flavonoids per day, equivalent to 500 g of vegetables, reduce the risk of colorectal cancer[332] by about 20%. For colon cancer, for a preventive and curative effect, it is necessary to favour fruits and vegetables rich in flavonols, i.e. onions, broccoli, spinach, cauliflowers, strawberries[332]. For rectal cancer, preference should be given to those rich in flavones such as celery, lettuce peppers, parsley, chervil, fennel and cabbage[332].

How to prevent and cure Crohn's disease

Crohn's disease is a chronic inflammatory bowel disease that can infect any part of the digestive system. It is a chronic disease that will manifest itself through diarrhea, abdominal pain or anal lesions. Although regarded as a rare disease, the number of new cases is increasing. There are currently about 3.5 million cases worldwide, mainly in Europe and the United States[333] [334]. Apart from genetic causes, environmental factors are very much involved: tobacco, disruption of the intestinal flora and food. It is quite possible to adopt preventive measures to prevent this disease. The first of these measures is smoking out[335]. The disease is increasingly manifesting itself in young women who have been exposed to stressful situations or the adoption of an industrial diet. Food additives used by industry can trigger Crohn's disease[336]. Products such as milk chocolates, ice creams, cheeses containing carrageenan (a thickener), can trigger the disease by destabilizing the intestinal immune system, especially if the food consumed per day provides more than 250 mg of this thickener[337]. Maltodextrin is an additive that serves as a flavouring, or to significantly increase the weight of the food. It is used in the composition of beers, cereal bars, chips... but is a destroyer of the intestinal flora[338]. Maintaining a good immune system, through a diet based on fruits and vegetables, is essential. The eviction of industrial power supply must be maximum. We have the case published in the journal Nutrients of June 2019, which describes the complete recovery of a 25-year-old man, thanks to a diet based on fruits and vegetables, after failure of traditional treatments[339].

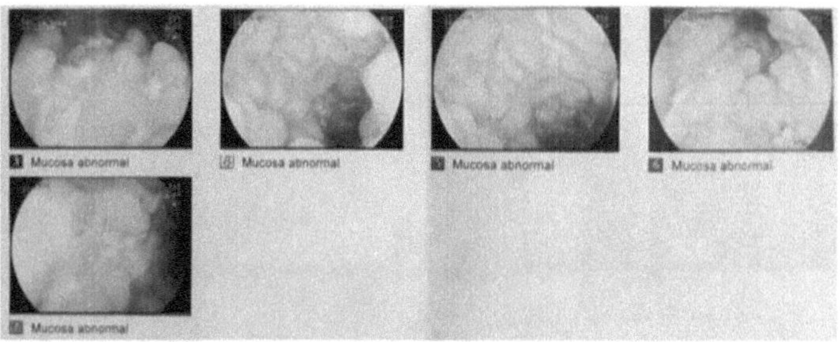

Colonoscopy images showing **ulcerations of the intestinal mucosa** of Crohn's disease at the time of diagnosis in 2014[339]. Creative Commons Crohn's Disease Remission with a Plant-Based Diet: A Case Report by https://www.mdpi.com/2072-6643/11/6/1385

After 2 years of drug infusion, and resumption of the disease, the young man and the medical team decided to completely eliminate the industrial diet based on meat, white flours and dairy products. The consumption of fruit and vegetables for 6 months alleviated the symptoms of the disease in 2017. The young man also practiced yoga and moderate intensity running. Until 2019, the patient no longer needs medication, and is stabilized just with his food made from fruits and vegetables.

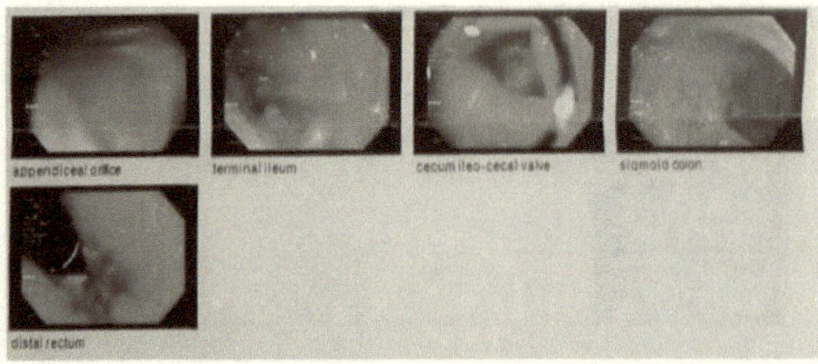

Colonoscopy images showing a disappearance of ulcerations of the intestinal mucosa of Crohn's disease, after 6 months of a diet rich in fruit and vegetables in 2017339. Creative Commons Crohn's Disease Remission with a Plant-Based Diet: A Case Report by https://www.mdpi.com/2072-6643/11/6/1385

A healthy diet can not only reverse the disease, but also prevent it from occurring. The diet must include fruit and vegetables to maintain the digestive flora by providing fibre. But be careful when the disease is declared, particular attention must be paid to the quality of the fibres consumed. For some patients, whole grain fibre should be avoided and the fibres of fruit and vegetables should be preferred.

How to prevent type 2 diabetes

Type 2 diabetes is currently booming worldwide. We are talking about an epidemic of diabetes. Type 1, which mainly affects children, is often linked to a genetic problem. For type 2, apart from cases also involving genetic factors, diet, lack of physical activity, sleep and weight are strongly involved. As mentioned above, acting on weight through diet and physical activity can significantly reduce the risk of type 2 diabetes. Reducing the BMI below 30 is a priority. For this, regular physical activity from 30 minutes to 1 hour a day is essential. Practicing daily walking is a quick solution: to do this, reduce car use, climb stairs, walk your dog, frequent a wooded park and get involved in work at home. For food, it is important to avoid industrial food, and to ensure a sufficient supply of fibre to maintain the digestive flora. Individuals who consume unprocessed whole grains throughout their lives reduce the risk of type 2 diabetes[340]; the important thing to know is that once the disease is diagnosed, it can be reversed by losing about 15% of the initial weight. For example, a person newly diagnosed with type 2 diabetes, who weighs 95 kg, can reverse the disease if he or she loses 14 kg. In studies in type 2 diabetics, a low-calorie diet for 3 to 6 months with weight loss ranging from 12 to 15 kg allows the pancreas to produce insulin again. To achieve these results, two phases are necessary. During Phase 1, on medical advice, patients should stop all drug treatments, and insulin injections, while following a very strict diet of 600-800 calories per day for two months. This phase allows an average weight loss of 14 kg. Then for 6 months (phase 2), patients must absolutely maintain the weight reduction obtained in phase 1, by following a diet that must remain stable (lower carbohydrates to 33%, increase protein to 33%, and maintain lipid intake to 33%). Under these conditions, 40% of diabetics had their blood sugar levels normalized by the end of Phase 2. Normal blood glucose levels were maintained for 6 months[341]. Significant weight loss is the key factor in reversing type 2 diabetes. By losing weight, the liver and pancreas also lose fat, which again allows better release and action of insulin in the pancreas and liver. Patients who lost more than 10 kg maintained the reversal of diabetes for 2 years. Patients are considered to have reversed their diabetes when they have long-term blood glucose levels (HbA1c) of less than 48 mmol/mol (<6.5%), without the need for type 2 diabetes medication[342]. These results are only possible if patients maintain the weight reduction at the level achieved at the end of the first phase, which can be extremely constraining for them. The failure rate is 75%. The question we ask ourselves is: are there other less painful methods to reverse diabetes? The answer is yes. The diet adopted after diagnosis is essential. As mentioned above, any diet that could induce the inflammatory process should be ruled out. In recent years, diets low in carbohydrates (low carb, 50 gr maximum carbohydrate per day), high in fat (70% fat) and balanced in protein (25%) have become popular in the management of several diseases, mainly obesity and diabetes[343].

Did you know? In the ketogenic or low carb diet, as carbohydrates are extremely limited, the body draws its necessary energy from the stock of muscles and liver. All carbohydrate-rich foods (bread, potatoes, chocolate, most fruits and vegetables, etc.) are discarded. In a first phase, we notice a significant weight loss. When the stock is depleted, the body naturally begins to use the lipids or fats provided by the diet in large proportions (more than 70%), with a production of waste called ketones. This diet can last for weeks or become a real way of eating.

However, studies report that these diets lead to increased mortality from cancer and cardiovascular disease[344][345][31]. And yet, the "Low carb" diet has led to significant weight reductions, with sometimes stopping anti-diabetic treatment in patients[346][347]. However, in the long term, the reduced intake of fibre and excess animal protein, together with saturated fatty acids, are extremely harmful and increase the mortality rate of patients[348][349]. The researchers deduce that to benefit from the "Low carb" diet, after the intensive weight loss phase, a sufficient fibre intake is necessary to avoid the side effects of this diet. Indeed, the consumption of whole grains (between 35 and 52 grams per day), which provide fibre, vitamins and trace elements, is necessary to reduce mortality in patients with chronic diseases[350][31]. For this reason, after the initial weight loss, it would be important to favour a long-term diet based on:

• Fruit, vegetables and whole grains rich in fibre (35 to 50 gr per day): avocados, broccoli, peppers, peppers, and carrots, blueberries, potatoes, pears, strawberries, flower choices, beans...

• Drink water before and during the meal (500 ml) to obtain a maximum swelling effect of the fibres.

• Unsaturated fatty acids: organic or wild salmon, sardines, walnut, olive or rapeseed oil.

• Vitamin B12: organic or wild salmon, sardines, tuna, mackerel, skinless poultry, mussels, oysters, clams, mackerel, herring, crabs...

Potatoes, peas and corn should be avoided as much as possible as they increase weight[45].

Prevent and naturally reverse brain diseases with omega-3, muscle irisin and natural melatonin

Neurodegenerative diseases could reach 100 million people worldwide by 2050[207]. Physical exercise, sleep and diet are the keys to their prevention. We must constantly keep in mind that the brain is the most fat-rich organ. It is necessary to provide it with good fatty acids for its construction and functioning. In the Middle Ages, Paracelsus, a Swiss doctor, formulated the theory of signatures, similia similibus curing which means "similar people heal similar people". The nut has all the appearance of a human brain, and is excellent for the brain. Eating nuts regularly, which provide a supply of omega-3, is essential to avoid deficiencies. A serving of 8 walnut kernels per day can improve sleep quality, learning and cognitive performance[351] [352]. If fats are part of the brain's building materials, sugar is its fuel. However, sugar consumption releases oxidizing molecules that accelerate brain aging over the years[353]. It is quite possible to slow down the destruction of neurons by consuming antioxidant molecules contained in fruits and vegetables. With blueberries, for example, which are rich in antioxidants, one cup a day increases memory, and improves learning abilities in Alzheimer's disease[354].

For most people, physical activity is involved in improving the heart's functions, while it impacts other organs, including the brain. Physical exercise releases endorphins into the bloodstream, which are "well-being" hormones. So far, various studies have shown that 150 minutes of physical activity per week improves memory and reduces the risk of Alzheimer's disease[355]. A hormone called irisin, released into the bloodstream by muscles during physical activity, promotes the neural growth of the brain's hippocampus by activating learning and memory[356]. Irisin is considered a real brain booster, thanks to physical activity.

In Parkinson's disease, a disease characterized by slowed movements, tremors, and motor rigidity, physical exercise by secretion of irisin has a neuro-protective effect, with less destruction of the motor neurons that control movement[357]. Thus, any individual who maintains regular physical exercise from the age of 50 or throughout his or her life reduces his or her risk of Parkinson's disease by 30%[358]. This is why one of the best strategies for the prevention and treatment of neurodegenerative diseases is the absolute necessity to move, play collective games, walk, practice dance, run, swim... As already mentioned, the respect of sleep-wake cycles, and the rhythm of melatonin secretion are important. Any deregulation of this hormone leads to neurodegenerative diseases, such as Parkinson's and Alzheimer's diseases. This is why sleep is a key factor in maintaining overall health. Looking back over the years, we have observed that drugs to fight Alzheimer's disease have been the subject of strong criticism for their effectiveness.

With regard to diet, the ketogenic diet has made it possible to slow the progression of Alzheimer's disease in some patients, provided that the early stages of the disease are addressed[359]. The striking fact is that, it is from the sixth week, with the appearance of ketone bodies, that the best results on memory appeared. The results also seem to improve motor skills in Parkinson's disease[360] [361].

However, great caution is needed for these 2 diseases, as the long-term results are not yet clear, especially since these diets lead to an increase in mortality from cancers and cardiovascular diseases[344] [345] [31]. In Alzheimer's disease, the consensus is that the brain is attacked by degeneration and inflammation. This results in amyloid plaques[362] and T proteins, forming neurofibrils and spreading to the entire brain[363]. The coexistence of amyloid plaques and the herpes virus observed in tissue samples suggest that this virus may be involved in the disease[364]. For Parkinson's disease, concerning dopamine deficiency in the brain, studies suggest that intestinal inflammation may be responsible for the disease in some patients[365]. Of all these elements, a diet based on antioxidants and fibre is necessary to counter neurodegenerative diseases.

How to prevent and treat cardiovascular disease:

Cardiovascular disease is the leading cause of death worldwide[366]. Potentially, it is cardiovascular diseases and their complications that pose the greatest threat to us. There is evidence that by adopting good lifestyle habits such as smoking cessation, healthy eating and physical exercise, we can prevent mortality from these diseases[367].

In any individual, the higher the volume of physical activity, the lower the risk of death from cardiovascular disease[368]. Anyone who spends 2000 calories per week reduces their cardiovascular mortality by 24%! For example, just taking 7500 steps, 5 days a week, allows us to achieve this objective. To remember 7500 steps a day, it is to spend 400 calories only by walking. Hence the importance of moving or practicing a sport regularly!

The second key point is the diet. While the impact of whole fruits and vegetables on cardiovascular mortality was considered very modest, a global study showed that eating too few fruits and vegetables kills millions of people each year through stroke or coronary heart disease[369]. The researchers explain that these are beneficial effects of fibres, flavonoids and carotenoids, through anti-inflammatory and antioxidant mechanisms, which significantly reduce "bad cholesterol", called LDL cholesterol, and restore the beneficial properties of "good cholesterol", called HDL cholesterol[370]. In addition, fruits and vegetables supply potassium on a daily basis, which has a protective role in cardiovascular disease, and more mainly in high blood pressure[371].

Researchers insist on the need to eat all fruits and vegetables in order to benefit from the very important benefits of fibre[372].

If there is one fruit I would advise you to adopt, it is the organic apple. Between waking up and the 10-hour break, find 5 minutes to enjoy one or two apples a day. You can vary with a pear, or a plum, or by adding a few nuts and almonds. The antioxidants contained in apples, especially in their skin, reduce cholesterol levels and the C-reactive protein that is a marker of inflammation. By introducing this habit, you automatically increase the chances that you won't need high blood pressure, or cholesterol medication for the rest of your life. By what mechanism? By consuming an apple daily for 6 months, there is a remarkable decrease in bad cholesterol of 23%, and an increase in good cholesterol of 4%[373]. The effect of atorvastatin 10 mg per day, one of the most prescribed cholesterol drugs, reduces bad cholesterol by 40% after 3 months[374]. With apples, not only is there an intake of 4 grams of fibre per day for the maintenance of the bacterial flora, but also the absence of adverse drug reactions.

I would also advise citrus fruits, and more particularly oranges, mandarins and clementines, which are easy to eat and for the presence of many flavonoids. I prefer them in the winter. A decrease in cardiovascular disease, and more particularly stroke related to atheromatous plaques, has been observed in Japanese people consuming citrus fruits once a day[375][287]. To ensure better efficacy against stroke, a minimum daily intake of vitamin B12 is necessary[37].

Nuts such as nuts contain polyunsaturated fatty acids, mainly omega-3 fatty acids and antioxidants. Regular consumption of nuts lowers bad cholesterol and reduces inflammation, while stimulating the immune system[376][377]. The consumption of one portion of nuts per day reduces cardiovascular disease by 37%[378]. In 2003, the FDA (Food and Drug Administration) encouraged the consumption of 43 g per day, of all kinds of nuts, for the reduction of cardiovascular disease. It is useful to remember that the nuts consumed must be unroasted, without salt or without added product. The consumption of fatty fish of ecological or wild origin (sardines, mackerel, salmon or herring...) containing fatty acids such as docosahexaeonic acid (DHA), and eicosapentaenoic acid (EPA), reduces the risk of myocardial infarction by reducing the formation of atheroma plaque[362]. To reduce coronary heart disease by 5%, it is necessary to consume 100 g of fish per week, or about 25 g, 4 times a week[379]. This risk reduction can be as high as 10% for stroke[380]. If the consumption of these products is too expensive for your budget, you should not hesitate to use rapeseed and olive oils for cooking and seasoning. Similarly, regular consumption of nuts is strongly recommended. Dietary supplements should be avoided as they do not guarantee the stability of omega-3[286]. Red fruits and vegetables containing lycopenes should also be part of the diet. Lycopenes are part of carotenoids, and are found in large quantities in tomatoes. They can also be found in watermelon, pumpkin, red pepper, grapes etc..... Regular consumption of whole products containing lycopenes reduces attacks of angina pectoris and myocardial infarction[381] [382]. This beneficial effect is explained by the reduction of bad cholesterol, and oxidative stress in the arteries[383] [384]. Berries (blackberries, blueberries, raspberries, strawberries...) are rich in flavonoids that reduce the risk of cardiovascular disease. They act mainly on inflammation and oxidative stress[385]. The consumption of a cup of fresh berries is sufficient to ensure a sufficient supply for one day.

The use of flavonoid-rich herbs and spices can reduce the consumption of cooking salts and fats. This is the case with saffron, which is known to contain crocin, a powerful antioxidant that reduces the formation of atheroma plaque[386]. Garlic is known to significantly reduce activity and rest blood pressure[387]. Do not hesitate to systematically add garlic to your meals.

For breakfast, systematically discard refined cereals, and prefer a whole grain such as oats. Regular consumption of whole grains, such as type 2[340] diabetes, reduces the risk of cardiovascular disease by 21%, thanks to the beneficial effect of fibre[388].

How to prevent osteo-articular diseases

Osteo-articular diseases are the second most debilitating diseases after mental illnesses[220]. They are mainly governed by an inflammatory process, except in the case of osteoporosis, which is characterized by a deterioration in the microarchitecture of bone tissue. Most people will talk about pain in a knee, fingers or back. As we have pointed out, these diseases do not only affect the elderly. Prevention is important, because when these diseases occur they are extremely painful. Everyone knows how back pain that doesn't go away can impact morale. The first rule is to quit smoking if you do, and to eat a healthy diet. All conditions that may promote deleterious factors, such as inflammation, should be gradually ruled out. Avoid weight gain because it increases the pressure on the joint cartilage and accelerates its destruction[389][390]. The maintenance of movements that relieve joints is necessary for prevention but also to treat pain, which occurs during these diseases. Non-traumatic stretching movements can be done at the end of the exercise sessions. If you are in pain, place a bag of moist heat on the sore spot for 10 minutes before you start exercising. Heat brings blood to the surface, reduces stiffness and sometimes relieves pain.

If you are taking pain medication, try to take it about 30 minutes before exercising to relieve yourself during stretching sessions.

1. **Protect the joints of both arms and neck by regularly stretching the pectoral and arm muscles (2 minutes)**

Stand at the entrance of a door, raise your right arm back and grasp the edge of the door with your right hand. Gently rotate the head to the left, and stay in this position for 15 to 30 seconds. And start again with the other arm.

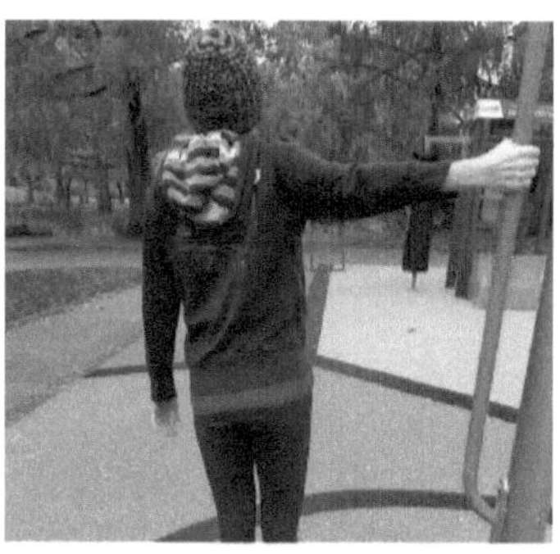

2. Protect knee and pelvic joints by regularly stretching hamstring muscles (5 minutes)

Hamstrings are the muscles located at the back of the thighs. In people who move little, these muscles are constantly contracted and eventually become stiff. However, it is these muscles that assure a good bending of the knees and pelvic movements. If stiff, knee and hip deflections cause severe pain.

Lying on your back, on a carpet or bed, bend your left knee and leave your left foot flat on the carpet or bed. Lift your right leg up in the air, and bend gently towards your chest, holding it with your hands. Hold this position for about 30 seconds, then release it slowly. Repeat this stretch on the left leg and then move on to the right leg.

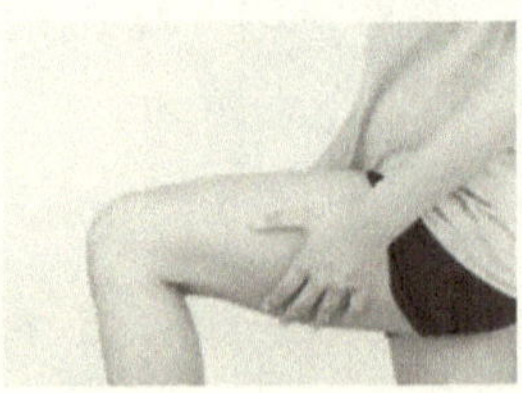

3. Protect the entire spine with the cat and cow (5 minutes)

- Sit on all fours, making sure that your hands are under your shoulders and your knees under your hips. Relax.
- On inspiration, dig your back by pushing your buttocks back and lifting your head. The back is then dug.

- On exhalation, round your back from the sacrum and finish with the cervicals. The back is then curved.
- Repeat the exercise 5 times as slowly as possible.

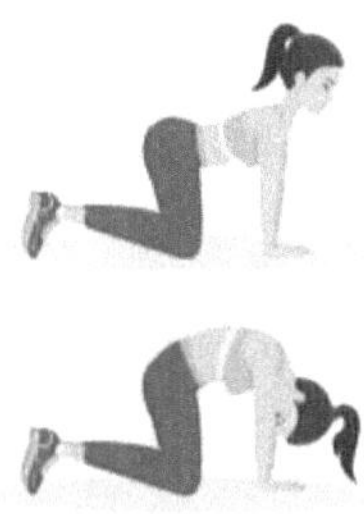

4. Protect foot joints by stretching calf muscles (2 minutes)

Stand in front of a wall, and lift yourself up on your toes. Hold the lift position for 30 seconds. Repeat 3 times.

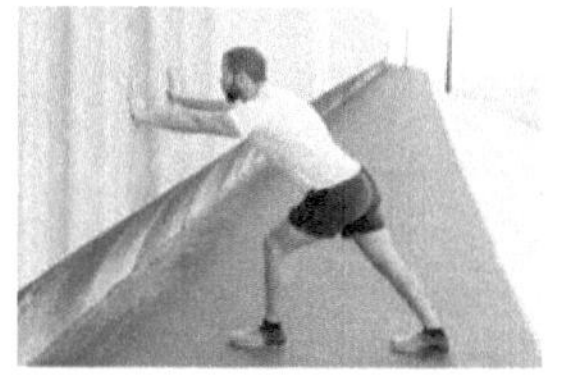

After these stretching examples, place an ice bag if you feel a painful area for about 5 minutes. Close your eyes and meditate if possible.

We have now reached the end of this book summarizing the essential points for pushing chronic diseases even further back. What to remember?

WEIGHT

<table>
<tr><td>✓</td><td>A diet containing at least 30 g of fibre per day (about 400 g of vegetables or fruit).</td></tr>
<tr><td>✓</td><td>Drink 2 x 125 ml glasses of water before and during each meal.</td></tr>
<tr><td>✓</td><td>Walk as much as possible, ideally 7500 steps a day, climb the stairs.</td></tr>
<tr><td>✓</td><td>10 minutes of scheduled morning exercises and 5 minutes of meditation (3 to 5 times a week).</td></tr>
<tr><td>✓</td><td>1 apple to chew between the alarm clock and the 10:00 break.</td></tr>
<tr><td>✓</td><td>Weekend end: get involved in housekeeping (15 minutes or more, walk in a wooded park).</td></tr>
<tr><td>✓</td><td>2 squares of dark chocolate in the morning around 10:00 am alternating with nuts.</td></tr>
</table>

STRESS

> ✓ 10 minutes of scheduled exercises in the morning and 5 minutes of meditation (3 to 5 times a week, see weights).
> ✓ Relax and listen to a short music you like.
> ✓ Watch or listen to comedy stories, keep in mind a story that always makes you laugh.
> ✓ 20 minutes of walking in the forest or wooded garden once a week (Saturday morning for example).

SLEEP

> ✓ Meditate regularly (e.g. after morning physical activities).
>
> ✓ Move, climb stairs, increase physical activity (see weights).
>
> ✓ Last coffee of the day before 2:00.

- ✓ Download filter applications that limit the effects of blue light.

- ✓ Do not use a screen for at least 1 hour before going to bed.

- ✓ Turn off the room screens or at worst disable all sound and vibration signals, relax.
- ✓ Go to bed at regular times.
- ✓ Respect the signs of sleepiness and fatigue (yawning and itchy eyes).
- ✓ Two one-hour naps a week, if necessary at weekends for example, to reduce cardiovascular risk.
- ✓ Healthy diet (see inflammation).
- ✓ Remember that it is sleep that cleanses the brain.

INFLAMMATION

✓ Maintain the balance of the intestinal flora by providing omega-3 fatty acids.
✓ 1 serving of 8 walnut kernels per day.
✓ 2 oils in your preparations: Olive oil for frying and rapeseed oil for seasoning.
✓ A diet rich in a variety of fruits and vegetables providing 30 g of fibre and at least 500 mg of flavonoids, or 400 g of vegetables and fruit per day.
✓ 20 minutes of walking 5 days a week: go up and down the stairs every day, don't take the car or walk to get to public transport if possible.

Finally, if you liked this book, please take the time to share your opinions, and post a positive review on Amazon. This is only the beginning of our common struggle for a better life. The best is yet to come!

AUTHOR BIOGRAPHY

David Friedman is a hospital pharmacist, with international skills in clinical pharmacy. He has saved countless lives and observed countless patients of all ages struggle with chronic disease.

He knows how costly and debilitating chronic disease can be, and this is why he spends hours of his free time reading the newest research on healthy nutrition, exercise, and other surprisingly effective methods of disease prevention.

As a pharmacist, he has first-hand knowledge of the risks and benefits of conventional medicine and the limitations of today's mainstream approaches to health. This is why he strongly advocates for preventive medicine that combines cutting-edge medical research with traditional techniques such as meditation.

David Friedman believes that health advice should be about motivation and empowerment to make healthy life choices, not about restrictions and unreasonable limits. He teaches flexible and realistic step-by-step strategies that help eliminate the key risk factors of most chronic diseases – without giving up on life's pleasures.

In his free time, David enjoys cooking and hiking in the woods with his family. His wife is a psychologist and meditation coach and his daughter wants to be a cancer researcher when she grows up.

BIBLIOGRAPHY

1. Wu, S. & hugo, A. Projection of Chronic Illness Prevalence and Cost Inflation. (2000).
2. Mortality and life expectancy statistics. (2017).
3. Ferlay, J. *et al.* Cancer incidence and mortality patterns in Europe: Estimates for 40 countries and 25 major cancers in 2018. *Eur. J. Cancer* **103**, 356–387 (2018).
4. Ferlay, J., Parkin, D. M. & Steliarova-Foucher, E. Estimates of cancer incidence and mortality in Europe in 2008. *Eur. J. Cancer* **46**, 765–781 (2010).
5. Shehab, N. *et al.* US Emergency Department Visits for Outpatient Adverse Drug Events, 2013-2014. *JAMA* **316**, 2115–2125 (2016).
6. How Bad is the Opioid Epidemic? *FRONTLINE* https://www.pbs.org/wgbh/frontline/article/how-bad-is-the-opioid-epidemic/.
7. Turque, B. Maryland governor declares state of emergency for opioid crisis. *Washington Post* (2017).
8. Jr, B. L. Fed chief Powell says the economic impact of the opioid crisis is 'quite substantial'. *CNBC* https://www.cnbc.com/2019/07/10/jerome-powell-says-economic-impact-of-opioid-crisis-is-substantial.html (2019).
9. Médicaments de la maladie d'Alzheimer : enfin non remboursables en France ! https://www.prescrire.org/fr/3/31/55116/0/NewsDetails.aspx.
10. Strelitz, J. *et al.* Changes in behaviors after diagnosis of type 2 diabetes and 10-year incidence of cardiovascular disease and mortality. *Cardiovasc Diabetol* **18**, 98 (2019).

11. Mirow, L. *et al.* [Recurrence of Crohn's disease after surgery--causes and risks]. *Zentralbl Chir* **133**, 182–187 (2008).
12. Kearney, P. M. *et al.* Global burden of hypertension: analysis of worldwide data. *Lancet* **365**, 217–223 (2005).
13. Rector, T. S., Anand, I. S. & Cohn, J. N. Relationships Between Clinical Assessments and Patients' Perceptions of the Effects of Heart Failure on Their Quality of Life. *Journal of Cardiac Failure* **12**, 87–92 (2006).
14. Lawes, C. M., Hoorn, S. V. & Rodgers, A. Global burden of blood-pressure-related disease, 2001. *The Lancet* **371**, 1513–1518 (2008).
15. Zhang, S. *et al.* Mushroom consumption and incident risk of prostate cancer in Japan: A pooled analysis of the Miyagi Cohort Study and the Ohsaki Cohort Study. *Int. J. Cancer* (2019) doi:10.1002/ijc.32591.
16. Aho, V. *et al.* Prolonged sleep restriction induces changes in pathways involved in cholesterol metabolism and inflammatory responses. *Sci Rep* **6**, 24828 (2016).
17. Obesity and overweight. https://www.who.int/news-room/fact-sheets/detail/obesity-and-overweight.
18. Hammond, R. A. & Levine, R. The economic impact of obesity in the United States. *Diabetes Metab Syndr Obes* **3**, 285–295 (2010).
19. Bhaskaran, K., Dos-Santos-Silva, I., Leon, D. A., Douglas, I. J. & Smeeth, L. Association of BMI with overall and cause-specific mortality: a population-based cohort study of 3·6 million adults in the UK. *Lancet Diabetes Endocrinol* **6**, 944–953 (2018).
20. Poirier, P. & Després, J.-P. Obésité et maladies cardiovasculaires. *Med Sci (Paris)* **19**, 943–949 (2003).
21. Grundy, S. M. Obesity, metabolic syndrome, and coronary atherosclerosis. *Circulation* **105**, 2696–2698 (2002).

22. Zhu, S. *et al.* Waist circumference and obesity-associated risk factors among whites in the third National Health and Nutrition Examination Survey: clinical action thresholds. *Am. J. Clin. Nutr.* **76**, 743–749 (2002).

23. Colditz, G. A., Willett, W. C., Rotnitzky, A. & Manson, J. E. Weight gain as a risk factor for clinical diabetes mellitus in women. *Ann. Intern. Med.* **122**, 481–486 (1995).

24. Zheng, Y. *et al.* Associations of Weight Gain From Early to Middle Adulthood With Major Health Outcomes Later in Life. *JAMA* **318**, 255–269 (2017).

25. Renehan, A. G., Tyson, M., Egger, M., Heller, R. F. & Zwahlen, M. Body-mass index and incidence of cancer: a systematic review and meta-analysis of prospective observational studies. *Lancet* **371**, 569–578 (2008).

26. Goodwin, P. J. *et al.* Insulin- and obesity-related variables in early-stage breast cancer: correlations and time course of prognostic associations. *J. Clin. Oncol.* **30**, 164–171 (2012).

27. Zhang, Y. *et al.* Angiopoietin-like protein 8 (betatrophin) is a stress-response protein that down-regulates expression of adipocyte triglyceride lipase. *Biochimica et Biophysica Acta (BBA) - Molecular and Cell Biology of Lipids* **1861**, 130–137 (2016).

28. Tobias, D. K. *et al.* Effect of low-fat diet interventions versus other diet interventions on long-term weight change in adults: a systematic review and meta-analysis. *Lancet Diabetes Endocrinol* **3**, 968–979 (2015).

29. Dyson, P. Low Carbohydrate Diets and Type 2 Diabetes: What is the Latest Evidence? *Diabetes Ther* **6**, 411–424 (2015).

30. Naude, C. E. *et al.* Low carbohydrate versus isoenergetic balanced diets for reducing weight and cardiovascular

risk: a systematic review and meta-analysis. *PLoS ONE* **9**, e100652 (2014).

31. Mazidi, M., Katsiki, N., Mikhailidis, D. P., Sattar, N. & Banach, M. Lower carbohydrate diets and all-cause and cause-specific mortality: a population-based cohort study and pooling of prospective studies. *Eur. Heart J.* **40**, 2870–2879 (2019).

32. Kaiser, K. A. *et al.* Increased fruit and vegetable intake has no discernible effect on weight loss: a systematic review and meta-analysis1234. *Am J Clin Nutr* **100**, 567–576 (2014).

33. Mytton, O. T., Nnoaham, K., Eyles, H., Scarborough, P. & Ni Mhurchu, C. Systematic review and meta-analysis of the effect of increased vegetable and fruit consumption on body weight and energy intake. *BMC Public Health* **14**, 886 (2014).

34. Pal, S., Khossousi, A., Binns, C., Dhaliwal, S. & Ellis, V. The effect of a fibre supplement compared to a healthy diet on body composition, lipids, glucose, insulin and other metabolic syndrome risk factors in overweight and obese individuals. *Br. J. Nutr.* **105**, 90–100 (2011).

35. Ma, Y. *et al.* Single-component versus multicomponent dietary goals for the metabolic syndrome: a randomized trial. *Ann. Intern. Med.* **162**, 248–257 (2015).

36. Ferdowsian, H. R. *et al.* A multicomponent intervention reduces body weight and cardiovascular risk at a GEICO corporate site. *Am J Health Promot* **24**, 384–387 (2010).

37. Tong, T. Y. N. *et al.* Risks of ischaemic heart disease and stroke in meat eaters, fish eaters, and vegetarians over 18 years of follow-up: results from the prospective EPIC-Oxford study. *BMJ* **366**, l4897 (2019).

38. Aguirre, M., Jonkers, D. M. A. E., Troost, F. J., Roeselers, G. & Venema, K. In vitro characterization of the impact of different substrates on metabolite

production, energy extraction and composition of gut microbiota from lean and obese subjects. *PLoS ONE* **9**, e113864 (2014).

39. Berding, K., Holscher, H. D., Arthur, A. E. & Donovan, S. M. Fecal microbiome composition and stability in 4- to 8-year old children is associated with dietary patterns and nutrient intake. *J. Nutr. Biochem.* **56**, 165–174 (2018).

40. Wassermann, B., Müller, H. & Berg, G. An Apple a Day: Which Bacteria Do We Eat With Organic and Conventional Apples? *Front Microbiol* **10**, (2019).

41. Rolls, B. J. Dietary energy density: Applying behavioural science to weight management. *Nutr Bull* **42**, 246–253 (2017).

42. Wanders, A. J. *et al.* Effects of dietary fibre on subjective appetite, energy intake and body weight: a systematic review of randomized controlled trials. *Obes Rev* **12**, 724–739 (2011).

43. Fulgoni, V. L., Dreher, M. & Davenport, A. J. Avocado consumption is associated with better diet quality and nutrient intake, and lower metabolic syndrome risk in US adults: results from the National Health and Nutrition Examination Survey (NHANES) 2001-2008. *Nutr J* **12**, 1 (2013).

44. Henning, S. M. *et al.* Hass Avocado Inclusion in a Weight-Loss Diet Supported Weight Loss and Altered Gut Microbiota: A 12-Week Randomized, Parallel-Controlled Trial. *Curr Dev Nutr* **3**, nzz068 (2019).

45. Bertoia, M. L. *et al.* Changes in Intake of Fruits and Vegetables and Weight Change in United States Men and Women Followed for Up to 24 Years: Analysis from Three Prospective Cohort Studies. *PLoS Med.* **12**, e1001878 (2015).

46. Van Walleghen, E. L., Orr, J. S., Gentile, C. L. & Davy, B. M. Pre-meal water consumption reduces meal energy

intake in older but not younger subjects. *Obesity (Silver Spring)* **15**, 93–99 (2007).

47. Dennis, E. A. *et al.* Water consumption increases weight loss during a hypocaloric diet intervention in middle-aged and older adults. *Obesity (Silver Spring)* **18**, 300–307 (2010).

48. Chazelas, E. *et al.* Sugary drink consumption and risk of cancer: results from NutriNet-Santé prospective cohort. *BMJ* **366**, l2408 (2019).

49. Ladabaum, U., Mannalithara, A., Myer, P. A. & Singh, G. Obesity, abdominal obesity, physical activity, and caloric intake in US adults: 1988 to 2010. *Am. J. Med.* **127**, 717-727.e12 (2014).

50. Matthews, C. E. *et al.* Amount of time spent in sedentary behaviors in the United States, 2003-2004. *Am. J. Epidemiol.* **167**, 875–881 (2008).

51. Saidj, M. *et al.* Descriptive study of sedentary behaviours in 35,444 French working adults: cross-sectional findings from the ACTI-Cités study. *BMC Public Health* **15**, 379 (2015).

52. 'Get Up!' or lose hours of your life every day, scientist says. *Los Angeles Times* https://www.latimes.com/science/sciencenow/la-sci-sn-get-up-20140731-story.html (2014).

53. Proper, K. I., Singh, A. S., van Mechelen, W. & Chinapaw, M. J. M. Sedentary behaviors and health outcomes among adults: a systematic review of prospective studies. *Am J Prev Med* **40**, 174–182 (2011).

54. Tremblay, M. S., Colley, R. C., Saunders, T. J., Healy, G. N. & Owen, N. Physiological and health implications of a sedentary lifestyle. *Appl Physiol Nutr Metab* **35**, 725–740 (2010).

55. Chau, J. Y. *et al.* Daily sitting time and all-cause mortality: a meta-analysis. *PLoS ONE* **8**, e80000 (2013).

56. Katzmarzyk, P. T. & Lee, I.-M. Sedentary behaviour and life expectancy in the USA: a cause-deleted life table analysis. *BMJ Open* **2**, (2012).

57. Lee, I.-M. *et al.* Association of Step Volume and Intensity With All-Cause Mortality in Older Women. *JAMA Intern Med* (2019) doi:10.1001/jamainternmed.2019.0899.

58. Bond Brill, J., Perry, A. C., Parker, L., Robinson, A. & Burnett, K. Dose-response effect of walking exercise on weight loss. How much is enough? *Int. J. Obes. Relat. Metab. Disord.* **26**, 1484–1493 (2002).

59. Oja, P. *et al.* Effects of frequency, intensity, duration and volume of walking interventions on CVD risk factors: a systematic review and meta-regression analysis of randomised controlled trials among inactive healthy adults. *Br J Sports Med* **52**, 769–775 (2018).

60. Murtagh, E. M. *et al.* The effect of walking on risk factors for cardiovascular disease: an updated systematic review and meta-analysis of randomised control trials. *Prev Med* **72**, 34–43 (2015).

61. Teh, K. C. & Aziz, A. R. Heart rate, oxygen uptake, and energy cost of ascending and descending the stairs. *Med Sci Sports Exerc* **34**, 695–699 (2002).

62. Jenkins, E. M., Nairn, L. N., Skelly, L. E., Little, J. P. & Gibala, M. J. Do stair climbing exercise 'snacks' improve cardiorespiratory fitness? *Appl Physiol Nutr Metab* **44**, 681–684 (2019).

63. Stamatakis, E. *et al.* Sitting Time, Physical Activity, and Risk of Mortality in Adults. *J. Am. Coll. Cardiol.* **73**, 2062–2072 (2019).

64. Cutt, H., Giles-Corti, B., Knuiman, M., Timperio, A. & Bull, F. Understanding dog owners' increased levels of physical activity: results from RESIDE. *Am J Public Health* **98**, 66–69 (2008).

65. Westgarth, C., Christley, R. M. & Christian, H. E. How might we increase physical activity through dog walking?: A comprehensive review of dog walking correlates. *Int J Behav Nutr Phys Act* **11**, (2014).

66. Knutson, K. L. & von Schantz, M. Associations between chronotype, morbidity and mortality in the UK Biobank cohort. *Chronobiol. Int.* **35**, 1045–1053 (2018).

67. Falcone, P. H. *et al.* Caloric expenditure of aerobic, resistance, or combined high-intensity interval training using a hydraulic resistance system in healthy men. *J Strength Cond Res* **29**, 779–785 (2015).

68. Schaun, G. Z., Pinto, S. S., Praia, A. B. de C. & Alberton, C. L. Energy expenditure and EPOC between water-based high-intensity interval training and moderate-intensity continuous training sessions in healthy women. *J Sports Sci* **36**, 2053–2060 (2018).

69. Adaptation of body protein metabolism in adult and aging man. - PubMed - NCBI. https://www.ncbi.nlm.nih.gov/pubmed/16829371.

70. Robinson, M. M. *et al.* Enhanced Protein Translation Underlies Improved Metabolic and Physical Adaptations to Different Exercise Training Modes in Young and Old Humans. *Cell Metabolism* **25**, 581–592 (2017).

71. Klika, B. & Jordan, C. HIGH-INTENSITY CIRCUIT TRAINING USING BODY WEIGHT: Maximum Results With Minimal Investment. *ACSM's Health & Fitness Journal* **17**, 8 (2013).

72. Viana, R. B. *et al.* Is interval training the magic bullet for fat loss? A systematic review and meta-analysis comparing moderate-intensity continuous training with high-intensity interval training (HIIT). *Br J Sports Med* **53**, 655–664 (2019).

73. Sultana, R. N., Sabag, A., Keating, S. E. & Johnson, N. A. The Effect of Low-Volume High-Intensity Interval

Training on Body Composition and Cardiorespiratory Fitness: A Systematic Review and Meta-Analysis. *Sports Med* (2019) doi:10.1007/s40279-019-01167-w.

74. pubmeddev & al, T. I., et. Effects of moderate-intensity endurance and high-intensity intermittent training on anaerobic capacity and VO2max. - PubMed - NCBI.

75. Horswill, C. A., Scott, H. M. & Voorhees, D. M. Effect of a novel workstation device on promoting non-exercise activity thermogenesis (NEAT). *Work* **58**, 447–454 (2017).

76. Differences of energy expenditure while sitting versus standing: A systematic review and meta-analysis - Farzane Saeidifard, Jose R Medina-Inojosa, Marta Supervia, Thomas P Olson, Virend K Somers, Patricia J Erwin, Francisco Lopez-Jimenez, 2018. https://journals.sagepub.com/doi/full/10.1177/204748731 7752186.

77. Health effects of sit-stand desks and interventions aimed to reduce sitting at work are still unproven. /news/health-effects-sit-stand-desks-and-interventions-aimed-reduce-sitting-work-are-still-unproven.

78. Reddy, S. The Price We Pay for Sitting Too Much. *Wall Street Journal* (2015).

79. Gregory, D. E. & Callaghan, J. P. Prolonged standing as a precursor for the development of low back discomfort: an investigation of possible mechanisms. *Gait Posture* **28**, 86–92 (2008).

80. Ekelund, U. *et al.* Dose-response associations between accelerometry measured physical activity and sedentary time and all cause mortality: systematic review and harmonised meta-analysis. *BMJ* **366**, l4570 (2019).

81. Steinberg, F. M., Bearden, M. M. & Keen, C. L. Cocoa and chocolate flavonoids: implications for cardiovascular health. *J Am Diet Assoc* **103**, 215–223 (2003).

82. Oliveira, D. & Nilsson, A. Effects of dark-chocolate on appetite variables and glucose tolerance: A 4 week randomised crossover intervention in healthy middle aged subjects. *Journal of Functional Foods* **37**, 390–399 (2017).

83. Massolt, E. T. *et al.* Appetite suppression through smelling of dark chocolate correlates with changes in ghrelin in young women. *Regul. Pept.* **161**, 81–86 (2010).

84. Marsh, C. E., Green, D. J., Naylor, L. H. & Guelfi, K. J. Consumption of dark chocolate attenuates subsequent food intake compared with milk and white chocolate in postmenopausal women. *Appetite* **116**, 544–551 (2017).

85. Tzounis, X. *et al.* Prebiotic evaluation of cocoa-derived flavanols in healthy humans by using a randomized, controlled, double-blind, crossover intervention study. *The American journal of clinical nutrition* **93**, 62–72 (2010).

86. Impact of intermittent fasting on health and disease processes. - PubMed - NCBI. https://www.ncbi.nlm.nih.gov/pubmed/27810402.

87. Harvie, M. *et al.* The effect of intermittent energy and carbohydrate restriction v. daily energy restriction on weight loss and metabolic disease risk markers in overweight women. *Br. J. Nutr.* **110**, 1534–1547 (2013).

88. Inc, G. Americans' Stress, Worry and Anger Intensified in 2018. *Gallup.com* https://news.gallup.com/poll/249098/americans-stress-worry-anger-intensified-2018.aspx.

89. Song, H. *et al.* Association of Stress-Related Disorders With Subsequent Autoimmune Disease. *JAMA* **319**, 2388–2400 (2018).

90. Bell, C. C. DSM-IV: Diagnostic and Statistical Manual of Mental Disorders. *JAMA* **272**, 828–829 (1994).

91. Brunet, A., Akerib, V. & Birmes, P. Don't throw out the baby with the bathwater (PTSD is not overdiagnosed). *Can J Psychiatry* **52**, 501–502; discussion 503 (2007).

92. Boscarino, J. A. Posttraumatic stress disorder and physical illness: results from clinical and epidemiologic studies. *Ann. N. Y. Acad. Sci.* **1032**, 141–153 (2004).

93. Boscarino, J. A., Forsberg, C. W. & Goldberg, J. A twin study of the association between PTSD symptoms and rheumatoid arthritis. *Psychosom Med* **72**, 481–486 (2010).

94. Yehuda, R., Teicher, M. H., Levengood, R. A., Trestman, R. L. & Siever, L. J. Circadian regulation of basal cortisol levels in posttraumatic stress disorder. *Ann. N. Y. Acad. Sci.* **746**, 378–380 (1994).

95. Passos, I. C. *et al.* Inflammatory markers in post-traumatic stress disorder: a systematic review, meta-analysis, and meta-regression. *Lancet Psychiatry* **2**, 1002–1012 (2015).

96. Shiga, H. *et al.* Life-event stress induced by the Great East Japan Earthquake was associated with relapse in ulcerative colitis but not Crohn's disease: a retrospective cohort study. *BMJ Open* **3**, e002294 (2013).

97. Remes, O., Brayne, C., van der Linde, R. & Lafortune, L. A systematic review of reviews on the prevalence of anxiety disorders in adult populations. *Brain Behav* **6**, e00497 (2016).

98. Negative emotions and acute physiological responses to stress. - PubMed - NCBI. https://www.ncbi.nlm.nih.gov/pubmed/10626027.

99. Cardiovascular differentiation of happiness, sadness, anger, and fear following imagery and exercise. - PubMed - NCBI.

100. Ekman, P. & Friesen, W. V. Felt, false, and miserable smiles. *J Nonverbal Behav* **6**, 238–252 (1982).

101.   Song, L., Che, W., Min-Wei, W., Murakami, Y. & Matsumoto, K. Impairment of the spatial learning and memory induced by learned helplessness and chronic mild stress. *Pharmacol. Biochem. Behav.* **83**, 186–193 (2006).

102.   Radley, J. J. *et al.* Chronic behavioral stress induces apical dendritic reorganization in pyramidal neurons of the medial prefrontal cortex. *Neuroscience* **125**, 1–6 (2004).

103.   Lupien, S. J., McEwen, B. S., Gunnar, M. R. & Heim, C. Effects of stress throughout the lifespan on the brain, behaviour and cognition. *Nat. Rev. Neurosci.* **10**, 434–445 (2009).

104.   Sarahian, N., Sahraei, H., Zardooz, H., Alibeik, H. & Sadeghi, B. Effect of Memantine Administration within the Nucleus Accumbens on Changes in Weight and Volume of the Brain and Adrenal Gland during Chronic Stress in Female Mice. in (2014).

105.   Echouffo-Tcheugui, J. B. *et al.* Circulating cortisol and cognitive and structural brain measures: The Framingham Heart Study. *Neurology* **91**, e1961–e1970 (2018).

106.   Gould, E., Tanapat, P., McEwen, B. S., Flügge, G. & Fuchs, E. Proliferation of granule cell precursors in the dentate gyrus of adult monkeys is diminished by stress. *PNAS* **95**, 3168–3171 (1998).

107.   Gould, E. & Tanapat, P. Stress and hippocampal neurogenesis. *Biol. Psychiatry* **46**, 1472–1479 (1999).

108.   Cole, G., Tucker, L. & Friedman, G. M. Relationships among measures of alcohol drinking behavior, life-events and perceived stress. *Psychol Rep* **67**, 587–591 (1990).

109.   stress-report.pdf.

110.   George, S. A., Khan, S., Briggs, H. & Abelson, J. L. CRH-stimulated cortisol release and food intake in healthy, non-obese adults. *Psychoneuroendocrinology* **35**, 607–612 (2010).

111.   Stress may add bite to appetite in women: a laboratory study of stress-induced cortisol and eating behavior. - PubMed - NCBI. https://www.ncbi.nlm.nih.gov/pubmed/11070333.

112.   Kirschbaum, C., Pirke, K. M. & Hellhammer, D. H. The 'Trier Social Stress Test'--a tool for investigating psychobiological stress responses in a laboratory setting. *Neuropsychobiology* **28**, 76–81 (1993).

113.   Chuang, J.-C. & Zigman, J. Ghrelin's Roles in Stress, Mood, and Anxiety Regulation. *International journal of peptides* **2010**, (2010).

114.   Dietary correlates of emotional eating in adolescence. - PubMed - NCBI. https://www.ncbi.nlm.nih.gov/pubmed/17466408.

115.   Anton, S. D. & Miller, P. M. Do negative emotions predict alcohol consumption, saturated fat intake, and physical activity in older adults? *Behav Modif* **29**, 677–688 (2005).

116.   Haedt-Matt, A. A. *et al.* Do emotional eating urges regulate affect? Concurrent and prospective associations and implications for risk models of binge eating. *Int J Eat Disord* **47**, 874–877 (2014).

117.   Cui, B. *et al.* Stress-induced epinephrine enhances lactate dehydrogenase A and promotes breast cancer stem-like cells. *J. Clin. Invest.* **129**, 1030–1046 (2019).

118.   Chiriac, V.-F., Baban, A. & Dumitrascu, D. L. Psychological stress and breast cancer incidence: a systematic review. *Clujul Med* **91**, 18–26 (2018).

119.   Song, H. *et al.* Perceived stress level and risk of cancer incidence in a Japanese population: the Japan

Public Health Center (JPHC)-based Prospective Study. *Sci Rep* **7**, 12964 (2017).

120. Kikuchi, N. *et al.* Perceived Stress and Colorectal Cancer Incidence: The Japan Collaborative Cohort Study. *Sci Rep* **7**, 40363 (2017).

121. Coleman, O. I. *et al.* Activated ATF6 Induces Intestinal Dysbiosis and Innate Immune Response to Promote Colorectal Tumorigenesis. *Gastroenterology* **155**, 1539-1552.e12 (2018).

122. Epel, E. S. *et al.* Accelerated telomere shortening in response to life stress. *Proc. Natl. Acad. Sci. U.S.A.* **101**, 17312–17315 (2004).

123. Coimbra, B. M., Carvalho, C. M., Moretti, P. N., Mello, M. F. & Belangero, S. I. Stress-related telomere length in children: A systematic review. *J Psychiatr Res* **92**, 47–54 (2017).

124. Puterman, E. *et al.* Lifespan adversity and later adulthood telomere length in the nationally representative US Health and Retirement Study. *Proc. Natl. Acad. Sci. U.S.A.* **113**, E6335–E6342 (2016).

125. Song, H. *et al.* Stress related disorders and risk of cardiovascular disease: population based, sibling controlled cohort study. *BMJ* **365**, l1255 (2019).

126. Wilbert-Lampen, U. *et al.* Cardiovascular events during World Cup soccer. *N. Engl. J. Med.* **358**, 475–483 (2008).

127. Kitamura, T., Kiyohara, K. & Iwami, T. The great east Japan earthquake and out-of-hospital cardiac arrest. *N. Engl. J. Med.* **369**, 2165–2167 (2013).

128. Type a behavior and your heart - American Journal of Cardiology. https://www.ajconline.org/article/0002-9149(75)90072-7/abstract.

129. Tawakol, A. *et al.* Relation between resting amygdalar activity and cardiovascular events: a

longitudinal and cohort study. *Lancet* **389**, 834–845 (2017).

130.   Chapotot, F., Buguet, A., Gronfier, C. & Brandenberger, G. Hypothalamo-pituitary-adrenal axis activity is related to the level of central arousal: effect of sleep deprivation on the association of high-frequency waking electroencephalogram with cortisol release. *Neuroendocrinology* **73**, 312–321 (2001).

131.   Atlantis, E., Chow, C.-M., Kirby, A. & Singh, M. F. An effective exercise-based intervention for improving mental health and quality of life measures: a randomized controlled trial. *Prev Med* **39**, 424–434 (2004).

132.   Singh, N. A., Clements, K. M. & Fiatarone, M. A. A randomized controlled trial of progressive resistance training in depressed elders. *J. Gerontol. A Biol. Sci. Med. Sci.* **52**, M27-35 (1997).

133.   Running versus weight lifting in the treatment of depression. - PubMed - NCBI. https://www.ncbi.nlm.nih.gov/pubmed/3454786.

134.   Cipriani, A. *et al.* Comparative efficacy and acceptability of 21 antidepressant drugs for the acute treatment of adults with major depressive disorder: a systematic review and network meta-analysis. *Lancet* **391**, 1357–1366 (2018).

135.   Hull, E. M., Young, S. H. & Ziegler, M. G. Aerobic fitness affects cardiovascular and catecholamine responses to stressors. *Psychophysiology* **21**, 353–360 (1984).

136.   Erickson, K. I. *et al.* Exercise training increases size of hippocampus and improves memory. *Proc Natl Acad Sci U S A* **108**, 3017–3022 (2011).

137.   Linnemann, A., Ditzen, B., Strahler, J., Doerr, J. M. & Nater, U. M. Music listening as a means of stress

reduction in daily life. *Psychoneuroendocrinology* **60**, 82–90 (2015).

138.   Ärzteblatt, D. Ä. G., Redaktion Deutsches. The Cardiovascular Effect of Musical Genres (20.05.2016). *Deutsches   Ärzteblatt* https://www.aerzteblatt.de/int/archive/article?id=179298.

139.   Anatomy   of   an   Illness. https://www.goodreads.com/work/best_book/179067-anatomy-of-an-illness-as-perceived-by-the-patient.

140.   Szabo, A., Ainsworth, S. E. & Danks, P. K. Experimental comparison of the psychological benefits of aerobic exercise, humor, and music. *Humor: International Journal of Humor Research* **18**, 235–246 (2005).

141.   Berk, L. S. *et al.* Neuroendocrine and stress hormone changes during mirthful laughter. *Am. J. Med. Sci.* **298**, 390–396 (1989).

142.   Yazdani, M., Esmaeilzadeh, M., Pahlavanzadeh, S. & Khaledi, F. The effect of laughter Yoga on general health among nursing students. *Iran J Nurs Midwifery Res* **19**, 36–40 (2014).

143.   Takahashi, K. *et al.* The elevation of natural killer cell activity induced by laughter in a crossover designed study. *Int. J. Mol. Med.* **8**, 645–650 (2001).

144.   Park, B. J., Tsunetsugu, Y., Kasetani, T., Kagawa, T. & Miyazaki, Y. The physiological effects of Shinrin-yoku (taking in the forest atmosphere or forest bathing): evidence from field experiments in 24 forests across Japan. *Environ Health Prev Med* **15**, 18–26 (2010).

145.   Li, Q. Effect of forest bathing trips on human immune function. *Environ Health Prev Med* **15**, 9–17 (2010).

146.   Hunter, M. R., Gillespie, B. W. & Chen, S. Y.-P. Urban Nature Experiences Reduce Stress in the Context

of Daily Life Based on Salivary Biomarkers. *Front Psychol* **10**, (2019).

147. Chen, K. W. *et al.* Meditative Therapies for Reducing Anxiety: A Systematic Review and Meta-analysis of Randomized Controlled Trials. *Depress Anxiety* **29**, 545–562 (2012).

148. Nidich, S. *et al.* Non-trauma-focused meditation versus exposure therapy in veterans with post-traumatic stress disorder: a randomised controlled trial. *Lancet Psychiatry* **5**, 975–986 (2018).

149. Kuyken, W. *et al.* Effectiveness and cost-effectiveness of mindfulness-based cognitive therapy compared with maintenance antidepressant treatment in the prevention of depressive relapse or recurrence (PREVENT): a randomised controlled trial. *Lancet* **386**, 63–73 (2015).

150. Hölzel, B. K. *et al.* Mindfulness practice leads to increases in regional brain gray matter density. *Psychiatry Res* **191**, 36–43 (2011).

151. Gotink, R. A., Meijboom, R., Vernooij, M. W., Smits, M. & Hunink, M. G. M. 8-week Mindfulness Based Stress Reduction induces brain changes similar to traditional long-term meditation practice - A systematic review. *Brain Cogn* **108**, 32–41 (2016).

152. Fuster, J. M. The prefrontal cortex--an update: time is of the essence. *Neuron* **30**, 319–333 (2001).

153. Hirshkowitz, M. *et al.* National Sleep Foundation's sleep time duration recommendations: methodology and results summary. *Sleep Health: Journal of the National Sleep Foundation* **1**, 40–43 (2015).

154. Liu, Y. Prevalence of Healthy Sleep Duration among Adults — United States, 2014. *MMWR Morb Mortal Wkly Rep* **65**, (2016).

155.   Beck, F., Richard, J.-B. & Léger, D. [Insomnia and total sleep time in France: prevalence and associated socio-demographic factors in a general population survey]. *Rev. Neurol. (Paris)* **169**, 956–964 (2013).

156.   Zhang, Y. *et al.* Worldwide and regional prevalence rates of co-occurrence of insomnia and insomnia symptoms with obstructive sleep apnea: A systematic review and meta-analysis. *Sleep Med Rev* **45**, 1–17 (2019).

157.   Hillman, D. *et al.* The economic cost of inadequate sleep. *Sleep* **41**, (2018).

158.   Hafner, M., Stepanek, M., Taylor, J., Troxel, W. M. & Van Stolk, C. Why sleep matters — the economic costs of insufficient sleep. https://www.rand.org/pubs/research_reports/RR1791.html (2016).

159.   Olfson, M., King, M. & Schoenbaum, M. Benzodiazepine use in the United States. *JAMA Psychiatry* **72**, 136–142 (2015).

160.   Kaufmann, C. N., Spira, A. P., Alexander, G. C., Rutkow, L. & Mojtabai, R. Trends in prescribing of sedative-hypnotic medications in the USA: 1993-2010. *Pharmacoepidemiol Drug Saf* **25**, 637–645 (2016).

161.   Edwards, B. A. *et al.* Aging and Sleep: Physiology and Pathophysiology. *Semin Respir Crit Care Med* **31**, 618–633 (2010).

162.   Hanlon, E. C. *et al.* Sleep Restriction Enhances the Daily Rhythm of Circulating Levels of Endocannabinoid 2-Arachidonoylglycerol. *Sleep* **39**, 653–664 (2016).

163.   Cappuccio, F. P. *et al.* Meta-analysis of short sleep duration and obesity in children and adults. *Sleep* **31**, 619–626 (2008).

164.   Yaggi, H. K., Araujo, A. B. & McKinlay, J. B. Sleep duration as a risk factor for the development of type 2 diabetes. *Diabetes Care* **29**, 657–661 (2006).
165.   Shan, Z. *et al.* Sleep Duration and Risk of Type 2 Diabetes: A Meta-analysis of Prospective Studies. *Diabetes Care* **38**, 529–537 (2015).
166.   Knutson, K. L. *et al.* Association between sleep and blood pressure in mid life: The CARDIA Sleep Study. *Arch Intern Med* **169**, 1055–1061 (2009).
167.   Aggarwal Brooke *et al.* Effects of Inadequate Sleep on Blood Pressure and Endothelial Inflammation in Women: Findings From the American Heart Association Go Red for Women Strategically Focused Research Network. *Journal of the American Heart Association* **7**, e008590 (2018).
168.   Ayas, N. T. *et al.* A prospective study of sleep duration and coronary heart disease in women. *Arch. Intern. Med.* **163**, 205–209 (2003).
169.   Larsson Susanna C. & Markus Hugh S. Genetic Liability to Insomnia and Cardiovascular Disease Risk. *Circulation* **140**, 796–798 (2019).
170.   Kojo, K., Pukkala, E. & Auvinen, A. Breast cancer risk among Finnish cabin attendants: a nested case-control study. *Occup Environ Med* **62**, 488–493 (2005).
171.   Altun, A. & Ugur-Altun, B. Melatonin: therapeutic and clinical utilization. *Int. J. Clin. Pract.* **61**, 835–845 (2007).
172.   McNeely, E. *et al.* Cancer prevalence among flight attendants compared to the general population. *Environmental Health* **17**, 49 (2018).
173.   Åkerstedt, T. *et al.* Sleep duration and mortality – Does weekend sleep matter? *Journal of Sleep Research* **28**, e12712 (2019).

174.   Häusler, N., Haba-Rubio, J., Heinzer, R. & Marques-Vidal, P. Association of napping with incident cardiovascular events in a prospective cohort study. *Heart* heartjnl-2019-314999 (2019) doi:10.1136/heartjnl-2019-314999.

175.   Hardeland, R. Antioxidative protection by melatonin: multiplicity of mechanisms from radical detoxification to radical avoidance. *Endocrine* **27**, 119–130 (2005).

176.   Blume, C., Garbazza, C. & Spitschan, M. Effects of light on human circadian rhythms, sleep and mood. *Somnologie (Berl)* **23**, 147–156 (2019).

177.   Russell, A. P. Molecular regulation of skeletal muscle mass. *Clin. Exp. Pharmacol. Physiol.* **37**, 378–384 (2010).

178.   Harfmann, B. D., Schroder, E. A. & Esser, K. A. Circadian rhythms, the molecular clock, and skeletal muscle. *J. Biol. Rhythms* **30**, 84–94 (2015).

179.   Chatterjee, S. & Ma, K. Circadian clock regulation of skeletal muscle growth and repair. *F1000Res* **5**, (2016).

180.   Cedernaes, J. *et al.* Acute Sleep Loss Induces Tissue-Specific Epigenetic and Transcriptional Alterations to Circadian Clock Genes in Men. *J. Clin. Endocrinol. Metab.* **100**, E1255-1261 (2015).

181.   Boelsma, E., Hendriks, H. F. & Roza, L. Nutritional skin care: health effects of micronutrients and fatty acids. *Am. J. Clin. Nutr.* **73**, 853–864 (2001).

182.   Oyetakin-White, P. *et al.* Does poor sleep quality affect skin ageing? *Clin. Exp. Dermatol.* **40**, 17–22 (2015).

183.   Kahan, V., Andersen, M. L., Tomimori, J. & Tufik, S. Can poor sleep affect skin integrity? *Med. Hypotheses* **75**, 535–537 (2010).

184.	Stress-induced changes in skin barrier function in healthy women. - PubMed - NCBI.

185.	Zhang, J. *et al.* Extended wakefulness: compromised metabolics in and degeneration of locus ceruleus neurons. *J. Neurosci.* **34**, 4418–4431 (2014).

186.	Benedict, C. *et al.* Acute sleep deprivation increases serum levels of neuron-specific enolase (NSE) and S100 calcium binding protein B (S-100B) in healthy young men. *Sleep* **37**, 195–198 (2014).

187.	Fultz, N. E. *et al.* Coupled electrophysiological, hemodynamic, and cerebrospinal fluid oscillations in human sleep. *Science* **366**, 628–631 (2019).

188.	Mechanisms of systems memory consolidation during sleep | Nature Neuroscience. https://www.nature.com/articles/s41593-019-0467-3.

189.	Wei, Y., Krishnan, G. P. & Bazhenov, M. Synaptic Mechanisms of Memory Consolidation during Sleep Slow Oscillations. *J. Neurosci.* **36**, 4231–4247 (2016).

190.	Studte, S., Bridger, E. & Mecklinger, A. Nap sleep preserves associative but not item memory performance. *Neurobiology of Learning and Memory* **120**, 84–93 (2015).

191.	Watson, N. F. *et al.* Transcriptional Signatures of Sleep Duration Discordance in Monozygotic Twins. *Sleep* **40**, (2017).

192.	Psychosocial and behavioral predictors of inflammation in middle-aged and older adults: the Chicago health, aging, and social relations study. - PubMed - NCBI.

193.	Prather, A. A. *et al.* Normative variation in self-reported sleep quality and sleep debt is associated with stimulated pro-inflammatory cytokine production. *Biol Psychol* **82**, 12–17 (2009).

194.   Friedman, E. M. *et al.* Social relationships, sleep quality, and interleukin-6 in aging women. *Proc. Natl. Acad. Sci. U.S.A.* **102**, 18757–18762 (2005).

195.   Burgos, I. *et al.* Increased nocturnal interleukin-6 excretion in patients with primary insomnia: a pilot study. *Brain Behav. Immun.* **20**, 246–253 (2006).

196.   Taylor, D. J., Kelly, K., Kohut, M. L. & Song, K.-S. Is Insomnia a Risk Factor for Decreased Influenza Vaccine Response? *Behav Sleep Med* **15**, 270–287 (2017).

197.   Banks, S., Van Dongen, H. P. A., Maislin, G. & Dinges, D. F. Neurobehavioral dynamics following chronic sleep restriction: dose-response effects of one night for recovery. *Sleep* **33**, 1013–1026 (2010).

198.   Belenky, G. *et al.* Patterns of performance degradation and restoration during sleep restriction and subsequent recovery: a sleep dose-response study. *J Sleep Res* **12**, 1–12 (2003).

199.   Ruiz, F. S. *et al.* Immune alterations after selective rapid eye movement or total sleep deprivation in healthy male volunteers. *Innate Immun* **18**, 44–54 (2012).

200.   Vgontzas, A. N. *et al.* Daytime napping after a night of sleep loss decreases sleepiness, improves performance, and causes beneficial changes in cortisol and interleukin-6 secretion. *Am. J. Physiol. Endocrinol. Metab.* **292**, E253-261 (2007).

201.   Faraut, B. *et al.* Napping reverses the salivary interleukin-6 and urinary norepinephrine changes induced by sleep restriction. *J. Clin. Endocrinol. Metab.* **100**, E416-426 (2015).

202.   Verster, J. C. & Koenig, J. Caffeine intake and its sources: A review of national representative studies. *Crit Rev Food Sci Nutr* **58**, 1250–1259 (2018).

203.   Elmenhorst, D., Meyer, P. T., Matusch, A., Winz, O. H. & Bauer, A. Caffeine occupancy of human cerebral A1 adenosine receptors: in vivo quantification with 18F-CPFPX and PET. *J. Nucl. Med.* **53**, 1723–1729 (2012).

204.   Drake, C., Roehrs, T., Shambroom, J. & Roth, T. Caffeine effects on sleep taken 0, 3, or 6 hours before going to bed. *J Clin Sleep Med* **9**, 1195–1200 (2013).

205.   Chang, A.-M., Aeschbach, D., Duffy, J. F. & Czeisler, C. A. Evening use of light-emitting eReaders negatively affects sleep, circadian timing, and next-morning alertness. *Proc. Natl. Acad. Sci. U.S.A.* **112**, 1232–1237 (2015).

206.   Wood, B., Rea, M. S., Plitnick, B. & Figueiro, M. G. Light level and duration of exposure determine the impact of self-luminous tablets on melatonin suppression. *Appl Ergon* **44**, 237–240 (2013).

207.   Ferri, C. P. *et al.* Global prevalence of dementia: a Delphi consensus study. *The Lancet* **366**, 2112–2117 (2005).

208.   Singh-Manoux, A. *et al.* Interleukin-6 and C-reactive protein as predictors of cognitive decline in late midlife. *Neurology* **83**, 486–493 (2014).

209.   Yaffe, K. *et al.* The metabolic syndrome, inflammation, and risk of cognitive decline. *JAMA* **292**, 2237–2242 (2004).

210.   Walker, K. A. *et al.* Systemic inflammation during midlife and cognitive change over 20 years: The ARIC Study. *Neurology* **92**, e1256–e1267 (2019).

211.   Cuello, A. C. Early and Late CNS Inflammation in Alzheimer's Disease: Two Extremes of a Continuum? *Trends Pharmacol. Sci.* **38**, 956–966 (2017).

212.   Villemagne, V. L. *et al.* Amyloid β deposition, neurodegeneration, and cognitive decline in sporadic

Alzheimer's disease: a prospective cohort study. *Lancet Neurol* **12**, 357–367 (2013).

213.   Wei, X. *et al.* Fatty acid synthesis configures the plasma membrane for inflammation in diabetes. *Nature* **539**, 294–298 (2016).

214.   Magalhaes, I. *et al.* Mucosal-associated invariant T cell alterations in obese and type 2 diabetic patients. *J. Clin. Invest.* **125**, 1752–1762 (2015).

215.   Taleb, S. Inflammation in atherosclerosis. *Arch Cardiovasc Dis* **109**, 708–715 (2016).

216.   Ross, R. & Harker, L. Hyperlipidemia and atherosclerosis. *Science* **193**, 1094–1100 (1976).

217.   Sabatine, M. S. *et al.* Evolocumab and Clinical Outcomes in Patients with Cardiovascular Disease. *N. Engl. J. Med.* **376**, 1713–1722 (2017).

218.   Sever, P. S. *et al.* Prevention of coronary and stroke events with atorvastatin in hypertensive patients who have average or lower-than-average cholesterol concentrations, in the Anglo-Scandinavian Cardiac Outcomes Trial--Lipid Lowering Arm (ASCOT-LLA): a multicentre randomised controlled trial. *Lancet* **361**, 1149–1158 (2003).

219.   Ridker, P. M. How Common Is Residual Inflammatory Risk? *Circ. Res.* **120**, 617–619 (2017).

220.   Woolf, A. D. Global burden of osteoarthritis and musculoskeletal diseases. *BMC Musculoskelet Disord* **16**, S3 (2015).

221.   McHugh, J. Epidemiology: Arthritis more common than expected. *Nature Reviews Rheumatology* **14**, 3–3 (2017).

222.   Wojdasiewicz, P., Poniatowski, Ł. A. & Szukiewicz, D. The role of inflammatory and anti-inflammatory cytokines in the pathogenesis of osteoarthritis. *Mediators Inflamm.* **2014**, 561459 (2014).

223.	Hootman, J. M., Helmick, C. G., Barbour, K. E., Theis, K. A. & Boring, M. A. Updated Projected Prevalence of Self-Reported Doctor-Diagnosed Arthritis and Arthritis-Attributable Activity Limitation Among US Adults, 2015–2040. *Arthritis Rheumatol* **68**, 1582–1587 (2016).

224.	Loftus, E. V. Clinical epidemiology of inflammatory bowel disease: Incidence, prevalence, and environmental influences. *Gastroenterology* **126**, 1504–1517 (2004).

225.	Bernstein, C. N. & Shanahan, F. Disorders of a modern lifestyle: reconciling the epidemiology of inflammatory bowel diseases. *Gut* **57**, 1185–1191 (2008).

226.	Ananthakrishnan, A. N. & Binion, D. G. Treatment of ulcerative colitis in the elderly. *Dig Dis* **27**, 327–334 (2009).

227.	Rohr, M. *et al.* Inflammatory Diseases of the Gut. *J Med Food* **21**, 113–126 (2018).

228.	van der Logt, E. M. J., Blokzijl, T., van der Meer, R., Faber, K. N. & Dijkstra, G. Westernized high-fat diet accelerates weight loss in dextran sulfate sodium-induced colitis in mice, which is further aggravated by supplementation of heme. *J. Nutr. Biochem.* **24**, 1159–1165 (2013).

229.	Gruber, L. *et al.* High fat diet accelerates pathogenesis of murine Crohn's disease-like ileitis independently of obesity. *PLoS ONE* **8**, e71661 (2013).

230.	Korolkova, O. Y., Myers, J. N., Pellom, S. T., Wang, L. & M'Koma, A. E. Characterization of Serum Cytokine Profile in Predominantly Colonic Inflammatory Bowel Disease to Delineate Ulcerative and Crohn's Colitides. *Clin Med Insights Gastroenterol* **8**, 29–44 (2015).

231.   Vollaard, E. J., Clasener, H. A., van Saene, H. K. & Muller, N. F. Effect on colonization resistance: an important criterion in selecting antibiotics. *DICP* **24**, 60–66 (1990).

232.   Saetta, M. *et al.* Activated T-lymphocytes and macrophages in bronchial mucosa of subjects with chronic bronchitis. *Am. Rev. Respir. Dis.* **147**, 301–306 (1993).

233.   Anthonisen, N. R., Connett, J. E. & Murray, R. P. Smoking and lung function of Lung Health Study participants after 11 years. *Am. J. Respir. Crit. Care Med.* **166**, 675–679 (2002).

234.   Waldmann, V. *et al.* [Sudden cardiac death: A better understanting for a better prevention]. *Ann Cardiol Angeiol (Paris)* **66**, 230–238 (2017).

235.   Di Franco, A. *et al.* Analysis of sputum cell counts during spontaneous moderate exacerbations of asthma in comparison to the stable phase. *J Asthma* **40**, 155–162 (2003).

236.   Fahy, J. V., Kim, K. W., Liu, J. & Boushey, H. A. Prominent neutrophilic inflammation in sputum from subjects with asthma exacerbation. *J. Allergy Clin. Immunol.* **95**, 843–852 (1995).

237.   Coyle, A. J. *et al.* Virus-specific CD8+ cells can switch to interleukin 5 production and induce airway eosinophilia. *J. Exp. Med.* **181**, 1229–1233 (1995).

238.   Multistage models of carcinogenesis. https://www.ncbi.nlm.nih.gov/pmc/articles/PMC1568502/ .

239.   Detection of chemical carcinogens by unscheduled DNA synthesis in rat liver primary cell cultures. - PubMed - NCBI. https://www.ncbi.nlm.nih.gov/pubmed/404038.

240.   Gomaa, E. A., Gray, J. I., Rabie, S., Lopez-Bote, C. & Booren, A. M. Polycyclic aromatic hydrocarbons in smoked food products and commercial liquid smoke flavourings. *Food Addit Contam* **10**, 503–521 (1993).

241.   Wang, X.-J. *et al.* Activation of Nrf2 by arsenite and monomethylarsonous acid is independent of Keap1-C151: enhanced Keap1-Cul3 interaction. *Toxicol. Appl. Pharmacol.* **230**, 383–389 (2008).

242.   Hussain, S. P. & Harris, C. C. Inflammation and cancer: an ancient link with novel potentials. *Int. J. Cancer* **121**, 2373–2380 (2007).

243.   Annunziata, C. M. *et al.* Frequent engagement of the classical and alternative NF-kappaB pathways by diverse genetic abnormalities in multiple myeloma. *Cancer Cell* **12**, 115–130 (2007).

244.   Lessard, L., Bégin, L. R., Gleave, M. E., Mes-Masson, A.-M. & Saad, F. Nuclear localisation of nuclear factor-kappaB transcription factors in prostate cancer: an immunohistochemical study. *Br. J. Cancer* **93**, 1019–1023 (2005).

245.   Bionaz, M., Hausman, G. J., Loor, J. J. & Mandard, S. Physiological and Nutritional Roles of PPAR across Species. *PPAR Res* **2013**, 807156 (2013).

246.   Jung, K. J. *et al.* Effect of short term calorie restriction on pro-inflammatory NF-kB and AP-1 in aged rat kidney. *Inflamm. Res.* **58**, 143–150 (2009).

247.   Rajendran, P. *et al.* Antioxidants and human diseases. *Clin. Chim. Acta* **436**, 332–347 (2014).

248.   Fernández-Sánchez, A. *et al.* Inflammation, oxidative stress, and obesity. *Int J Mol Sci* **12**, 3117–3132 (2011).

249.   Herieka, M. & Erridge, C. High-fat meal induced postprandial inflammation. *Mol Nutr Food Res* **58**, 136–146 (2014).

250.   Jansen, F. *et al.* High glucose condition increases NADPH oxidase activity in endothelial microparticles that promote vascular inflammation. *Cardiovasc. Res.* **98**, 94–106 (2013).

251.   Miller, J. B., Pang, E. & Bramall, L. Rice: a high or low glycemic index food? *Am. J. Clin. Nutr.* **56**, 1034–1036 (1992).

252.   Hu, E. A., Pan, A., Malik, V. & Sun, Q. White rice consumption and risk of type 2 diabetes: meta-analysis and systematic review. *BMJ* **344**, e1454 (2012).

253.   Sun, Q. *et al.* White rice, brown rice, and risk of type 2 diabetes in US men and women. *Arch. Intern. Med.* **170**, 961–969 (2010).

254.   Park, J. *et al.* Increase in glucose-6-phosphate dehydrogenase in adipocytes stimulates oxidative stress and inflammatory signals. *Diabetes* **55**, 2939–2949 (2006).

255.   Elmarakby, A. A. & Sullivan, J. C. Relationship between oxidative stress and inflammatory cytokines in diabetic nephropathy. *Cardiovasc Ther* **30**, 49–59 (2012).

256.   DiNicolantonio, J. J., O'Keefe, J. H. & Lucan, S. C. Added fructose: a principal driver of type 2 diabetes mellitus and its consequences. *Mayo Clin. Proc.* **90**, 372–381 (2015).

257.   Hu, F. B. & Malik, V. S. Sugar-sweetened beverages and risk of obesity and type 2 diabetes: epidemiologic evidence. *Physiol. Behav.* **100**, 47–54 (2010).

258.   Karl, J. P. *et al.* Substituting whole grains for refined grains in a 6-wk randomized trial favorably affects energy-balance metrics in healthy men and postmenopausal women. *Am. J. Clin. Nutr.* **105**, 589–599 (2017).

259.   Wang, Y. *et al.* Whole grain and cereal fiber intake and the risk of type 2 diabetes: a meta-analysis. *Int J Mol Epidemiol Genet* **10**, 38–46 (2019).

260.   Monguchi, T. *et al.* Excessive intake of trans fatty acid accelerates atherosclerosis through promoting inflammation and oxidative stress in a mouse model of hyperlipidemia. *J Cardiol* **70**, 121–127 (2017).

261.   Wang, Q. *et al.* Impact of Nonoptimal Intakes of Saturated, Polyunsaturated, and Trans Fat on Global Burdens of Coronary Heart Disease. *J Am Heart Assoc* **5**, (2016).

262.   Astiasarán, I., Abella, E., Gatta, G. & Ansorena, D. Margarines and Fast-Food French Fries: Low Content of trans Fatty Acids. *Nutrients* **9**, (2017).

263.   Nishida, C. & Uauy, R. WHO Scientific Update on health consequences of trans fatty acids: introduction. *Eur J Clin Nutr* **63 Suppl 2**, S1-4 (2009).

264.   Contamination of meat products during smoking by polycyclic aromatic hydrocarbons: Processes and Prevention | Request PDF. https://www.researchgate.net/publication/282299360_Co ntamination_of_meat_products_during_smoking_by_poly cyclic_aromatic_hydrocarbons_Processes_and_Preventio n.

265.   Van Hecke, T. *et al.* Increased oxidative and nitrosative reactions during digestion could contribute to the association between well-done red meat consumption and colorectal cancer. *Food Chem* **187**, 29–36 (2015).

266.   IARC Monographs evaluate consumption of red meat and processed meat. 2.

267.   Huang, S. *et al.* Saturated fatty acids activate TLR-mediated proinflammatory signaling pathways. *J. Lipid Res.* **53**, 2002–2013 (2012).

268.   Rioux, V. & Legrand, P. Saturated fatty acids: simple molecular structures with complex cellular functions. *Curr Opin Clin Nutr Metab Care* **10**, 752–758 (2007).

269.   Bruce, K. D. *et al.* Maternal high-fat feeding primes steatohepatitis in adult mice offspring, involving mitochondrial dysfunction and altered lipogenesis gene expression. *Hepatology* **50**, 1796–1808 (2009).

270.   Ballal, K., Wilson, C. R., Harmancey, R. & Taegtmeyer, H. Obesogenic High Fat Western Diet Induces Oxidative Stress and Apoptosis in Rat Heart. *Mol Cell Biochem* **344**, 221–230 (2010).

271.   Anderson, E. J. *et al.* Mitochondrial H2O2 emission and cellular redox state link excess fat intake to insulin resistance in both rodents and humans. *J. Clin. Invest.* **119**, 573–581 (2009).

272.   Virgin Olive Oil and Health: Summary of the III International Conference on Virgin Olive Oil and Health Consensus Report, JAEN (Spain) 2018. https://www.ncbi.nlm.nih.gov/pmc/articles/PMC6770785/
.

273.   Yu, K. S., Cho, H. & Hwang, K. T. Physicochemical properties and oxidative stability of frying oils during repeated frying of potato chips. *Food Sci. Biotechnol.* **27**, 651–659 (2018).

274.   Macpherson, A. J., Hunziker, L., McCoy, K. & Lamarre, A. IgA responses in the intestinal mucosa against pathogenic and non-pathogenic microorganisms. *Microbes Infect.* **3**, 1021–1035 (2001).

275.   Bauer, H., Horowitz, R. E., Levenson, S. M. & Popper, H. The response of the lymphatic tissue to the microbial flora. Studies on germfree mice. *Am. J. Pathol.* **42**, 471–483 (1963).

276.	Miquel, S. *et al.* Identification of metabolic signatures linked to anti-inflammatory effects of Faecalibacterium prausnitzii. *MBio* **6**, (2015).
277.	Lopetuso, L. R. *et al.* The therapeutic management of gut barrier leaking: the emerging role for mucosal barrier protectors. *Eur Rev Med Pharmacol Sci* **19**, 1068–1076 (2015).
278.	Jiang, C., Li, G., Huang, P., Liu, Z. & Zhao, B. The Gut Microbiota and Alzheimer's Disease. *J. Alzheimers Dis.* **58**, 1–15 (2017).
279.	Gao, R., Gao, Z., Huang, L. & Qin, H. Gut microbiota and colorectal cancer. *Eur. J. Clin. Microbiol. Infect. Dis.* **36**, 757–769 (2017).
280.	Simopoulos, A. P. An Increase in the Omega-6/Omega-3 Fatty Acid Ratio Increases the Risk for Obesity. *Nutrients* **8**, (2016).
281.	Menni, C. *et al.* Omega-3 fatty acids correlate with gut microbiome diversity and production of N-carbamylglutamate in middle aged and elderly women. *Sci Rep* **7**, 1–11 (2017).
282.	Kris-Etherton, P. M., Harris, W. S., Appel, L. J. & American Heart Association. Nutrition Committee. Fish consumption, fish oil, omega-3 fatty acids, and cardiovascular disease. *Circulation* **106**, 2747–2757 (2002).
283.	Simopoulos, A. P. The importance of the omega-6/omega-3 fatty acid ratio in cardiovascular disease and other chronic diseases. *Exp. Biol. Med. (Maywood)* **233**, 674–688 (2008).
284.	Kiecolt-Glaser, J. K., Belury, M. A., Andridge, R., Malarkey, W. B. & Glaser, R. Omega-3 supplementation lowers inflammation and anxiety in medical students: a randomized controlled trial. *Brain Behav. Immun.* **25**, 1725–1734 (2011).

285.   Abdelhamid, A. S. *et al.* Omega-3 fatty acids for the primary and secondary prevention of cardiovascular disease. *Cochrane Database Syst Rev* **11**, CD003177 (2018).

286.   Jackowski, S. A. *et al.* Oxidation levels of North American over-the-counter n-3 (omega-3) supplements and the influence of supplement formulation and delivery form on evaluating oxidative safety. *J Nutr Sci* **4**, e30 (2015).

287.   Bondonno, N. P. *et al.* Flavonoid intake is associated with lower mortality in the Danish Diet Cancer and Health Cohort. *Nat Commun* **10**, 3651 (2019).

288.   Ruiz, P. A. & Haller, D. Functional diversity of flavonoids in the inhibition of the proinflammatory NF-kappaB, IRF, and Akt signaling pathways in murine intestinal epithelial cells. *J. Nutr.* **136**, 664–671 (2006).

289.   Cuadrado, A., Martín-Moldes, Z., Ye, J. & Lastres-Becker, I. Transcription factors NRF2 and NF-κB are coordinated effectors of the Rho family, GTP-binding protein RAC1 during inflammation. *J. Biol. Chem.* **289**, 15244–15258 (2014).

290.   Dietary Flavonoids and Colorectal Adenoma Recurrence in the Polyp Prevention Trial. https://www.ncbi.nlm.nih.gov/pmc/articles/PMC2517243/

291.   Bobe, G. *et al.* Serum cytokine concentrations, flavonol intake and colorectal adenoma recurrence in the Polyp Prevention Trial. *Br. J. Cancer* **103**, 1453–1461 (2010).

292.   Inflammation and exercise: Inhibition of monocytic intracellular TNF production by acute exercise via β2-adrenergic activation. - PubMed - NCBI. https://www.ncbi.nlm.nih.gov/pubmed/28011264.

293.   Pedersen, B. K. Anti-inflammatory effects of exercise: role in diabetes and cardiovascular disease. *Eur. J. Clin. Invest.* **47**, 600–611 (2017).
294.   Peto, R., Lopez, A. D., Boreham, J., Thun, M. & Heath, C. Mortality from tobacco in developed countries: indirect estimation from national vital statistics. *Lancet* **339**, 1268–1278 (1992).
295.   Bade, B. C., Thomas, D. D., Scott, J. B. & Silvestri, G. A. Increasing physical activity and exercise in lung cancer: reviewing safety, benefits, and application. *J Thorac Oncol* **10**, 861–871 (2015).
296.   Divisi, D., Di Francesco, C., Di Leonardo, G. & Crisci, R. Preoperative pulmonary rehabilitation in patients with lung cancer and chronic obstructive pulmonary disease. *Eur J Cardiothorac Surg* **43**, 293–296 (2013).
297.   Bobbio, A. *et al.* Preoperative pulmonary rehabilitation in patients undergoing lung resection for non-small cell lung cancer. *Eur J Cardiothorac Surg* **33**, 95–98 (2008).
298.   Lin, Y.-Y., Liu, M. F., Tzeng, J.-I. & Lin, C.-C. Effects of Walking on Quality of Life Among Lung Cancer Patients: A Longitudinal Study. *Cancer Nurs* **38**, 253–259 (2015).
299.   Warburton, D. E. R., Nicol, C. W. & Bredin, S. S. D. Health benefits of physical activity: the evidence. *CMAJ* **174**, 801–809 (2006).
300.   Hung, R. *et al.* Fatigue and Functional Impairment in Early-Stage Non-Small Cell Lung Cancer Survivors. *J Pain Symptom Manage* **41**, 426–435 (2011).
301.   McTiernan, A. Mechanisms linking physical activity with cancer. *Nat. Rev. Cancer* **8**, 205–211 (2008).
302.   Büchner, F. L. *et al.* Variety in fruit and vegetable consumption and the risk of lung cancer in the European

prospective investigation into cancer and nutrition. *Cancer Epidemiol. Biomarkers Prev.* **19**, 2278–2286 (2010).

303.   Vieira, A. R. *et al.* Fruits, vegetables and lung cancer risk: a systematic review and meta-analysis. *Ann. Oncol.* **27**, 81–96 (2016).

304.   Albanes, D. *et al.* Alpha-Tocopherol and beta-carotene supplements and lung cancer incidence in the alpha-tocopherol, beta-carotene cancer prevention study: effects of base-line characteristics and study compliance. *J. Natl. Cancer Inst.* **88**, 1560–1570 (1996).

305.   Bray, F. *et al.* Global cancer statistics 2018: GLOBOCAN estimates of incidence and mortality worldwide for 36 cancers in 185 countries. *CA Cancer J Clin* **68**, 394–424 (2018).

306.   Sinclair, J. *et al.* The acceptability of addressing alcohol consumption as a modifiable risk factor for breast cancer: a mixed method study within breast screening services and symptomatic breast clinics. *BMJ Open* **9**, e027371 (2019).

307.   Lee, I.-M. Physical activity and cancer prevention--data from epidemiologic studies. *Med Sci Sports Exerc* **35**, 1823–1827 (2003).

308.   Effect of Physical Activity on Women at Increased Risk of Breast Cancer: Results from the E3N Cohort Study | Cancer Epidemiology, Biomarkers & Prevention. https://cebp.aacrjournals.org/content/15/1/57.

309.   McTiernan, A. *et al.* Effect of exercise on serum estrogens in postmenopausal women: a 12-month randomized clinical trial. *Cancer Res.* **64**, 2923–2928 (2004).

310.   Lahart, I. M., Metsios, G. S., Nevill, A. M. & Carmichael, A. R. Physical activity for women with

breast cancer after adjuvant therapy. *Cochrane Database Syst Rev* **2018**, (2018).
311.   Furmaniak, A. C., Menig, M. & Markes, M. H. Exercise for women receiving adjuvant therapy for breast cancer. *Cochrane Database Syst Rev* **2016**, (2016).
312.   Jones, M. E., Schoemaker, M. J., Wright, L. B., Ashworth, A. & Swerdlow, A. J. Smoking and risk of breast cancer in the Generations Study cohort. *Breast Cancer Res* **19**, (2017).
313.   Farvid, M. S. *et al.* Fruit and vegetable consumption and breast cancer incidence: Repeated measures over 30 years of follow-up. *Int. J. Cancer* **144**, 1496–1510 (2019).
314.   Demark-Wahnefried, W., Campbell, K. L. & Hayes, S. C. Weight management and its role in breast cancer rehabilitation. *Cancer* **118**, 2277–2287 (2012).
315.   Knott, S. R. V. *et al.* Asparagine bioavailability governs metastasis in a model of breast cancer. *Nature* **554**, 378–381 (2018).
316.   Prostate cancer | Nature. https://www.nature.com/articles/528S117a.
317.   Johnsen, N. F. *et al.* Physical activity and risk of prostate cancer in the European Prospective Investigation into Cancer and Nutrition (EPIC) cohort. *Int. J. Cancer* **125**, 902–908 (2009).
318.   Patel, A. V. *et al.* Recreational physical activity and risk of prostate cancer in a large cohort of U.S. men. *Cancer Epidemiol. Biomarkers Prev.* **14**, 275–279 (2005).
319.   Friedenreich, C. M. *et al.* Physical Activity and Survival After Prostate Cancer. *Eur. Urol.* **70**, 576–585 (2016).
320.   Ahn, J. *et al.* Dairy products, calcium intake, and risk of prostate cancer in the prostate, lung, colorectal, and ovarian cancer screening trial. *Cancer Epidemiol. Biomarkers Prev.* **16**, 2623–2630 (2007).

321.   Brasky, T. M. *et al.* Plasma Phospholipid Fatty Acids and Prostate Cancer Risk in the SELECT Trial. *J Natl Cancer Inst* **105**, 1132–1141 (2013).

322.   Boland, C. R., Luciani, M. G., Gasche, C. & Goel, A. INFECTION, INFLAMMATION, AND GASTROINTESTINAL CANCER. *Gut* **54**, 1321–1331 (2005).

323.   Nagini, S. Carcinoma of the stomach: A review of epidemiology, pathogenesis, molecular genetics and chemoprevention. *World J Gastrointest Oncol* **4**, 156–169 (2012).

324.   Sanchez, N. F. *et al.* Physical activity reduces risk for colon polyps in a multiethnic colorectal cancer screening population. *BMC Res Notes* **5**, 312 (2012).

325.   Baltgalvis, K. A., Berger, F. G., Peña, M. M. O., Davis, J. M. & Carson, J. A. The interaction of a high-fat diet and regular moderate intensity exercise on intestinal polyp development in Apc Min/+ mice. *Cancer Prev Res (Phila)* **2**, 641–649 (2009).

326.   Chao, A. *et al.* Amount, type, and timing of recreational physical activity in relation to colon and rectal cancer in older adults: the Cancer Prevention Study II Nutrition Cohort. *Cancer Epidemiol. Biomarkers Prev.* **13**, 2187–2195 (2004).

327.   Thune, I. & Furberg, A. S. Physical activity and cancer risk: dose-response and cancer, all sites and site-specific. *Med Sci Sports Exerc* **33**, S530-550; discussion S609-610 (2001).

328.   Halle, M. & Schoenberg, M. H. Physical activity in the prevention and treatment of colorectal carcinoma. *Dtsch Arztebl Int* **106**, 722–727 (2009).

329.   Cho, E. *et al.* Dairy foods, calcium, and colorectal cancer: a pooled analysis of 10 cohort studies. *J. Natl. Cancer Inst.* **96**, 1015–1022 (2004).

330.   O'Keefe, S. J. D. *et al.* Fat, fibre and cancer risk in African Americans and rural Africans. *Nat Commun* **6**, 6342 (2015).

331.   Song, M. *et al.* Fiber Intake and Survival After Colorectal Cancer Diagnosis. *JAMA Oncol* **4**, 71–79 (2018).

332.   Chang, H., Lei, L., Zhou, Y., Ye, F. & Zhao, G. Dietary Flavonoids and the Risk of Colorectal Cancer: An Updated Meta-Analysis of Epidemiological Studies. *Nutrients* **10**, (2018).

333.   Ng, S. C. *et al.* Worldwide incidence and prevalence of inflammatory bowel disease in the 21st century: a systematic review of population-based studies. *Lancet* **390**, 2769–2778 (2018).

334.   Kappelman, M. D., Moore, K. R., Allen, J. K. & Cook, S. F. Recent Trends in the Prevalence of Crohn's Disease and Ulcerative Colitis in a Commercially Insured US Population. *Dig Dis Sci* **58**, 519–525 (2013).

335.   Seksik, P., Nion-Larmurier, I., Sokol, H., Beaugerie, L. & Cosnes, J. Effects of light smoking consumption on the clinical course of Crohn's disease. *Inflamm. Bowel Dis.* **15**, 734–741 (2009).

336.   Kakodkar, S. & Mutlu, E. A. Diet as a therapeutic option for adult inflammatory bowel disease. *Gastroenterol Clin North Am* **46**, 745–767 (2017).

337.   Tobacman, J. K. Review of harmful gastrointestinal effects of carrageenan in animal experiments. *Environ. Health Perspect.* **109**, 983–994 (2001).

338.   Nickerson, K. P., Chanin, R. & McDonald, C. Deregulation of intestinal anti-microbial defense by the dietary additive, maltodextrin. *Gut Microbes* **6**, 78–83 (2015).

339.   Sandefur, K., Kahleova, H., Desmond, A. N., Elfrink, E. & Barnard, N. D. Crohn's Disease Remission

with a Plant-Based Diet: A Case Report. *Nutrients* **11**, (2019).

340. Riccardi, G., Capaldo, B. & Vaccaro, O. Functional foods in the management of obesity and type 2 diabetes. *Curr Opin Clin Nutr Metab Care* **8**, 630–635 (2005).

341. Steven, S. *et al.* Very Low-Calorie Diet and 6 Months of Weight Stability in Type 2 Diabetes: Pathophysiological Changes in Responders and Nonresponders. *Diabetes Care* **39**, 808–815 (2016).

342. Durability of a primary care-led weight-management intervention for remission of type 2 diabetes: 2-year results of the DiRECT open-label, cluster-... - PubMed - NCBI. https://www.ncbi.nlm.nih.gov/pubmed/30852132.

343. Clifton, P. M., Condo, D. & Keogh, J. B. Long term weight maintenance after advice to consume low carbohydrate, higher protein diets--a systematic review and meta analysis. *Nutr Metab Cardiovasc Dis* **24**, 224–235 (2014).

344. Santos, F. L., Esteves, S. S., da Costa Pereira, A., Yancy, W. S. & Nunes, J. P. L. Systematic review and meta-analysis of clinical trials of the effects of low carbohydrate diets on cardiovascular risk factors. *Obes Rev* **13**, 1048–1066 (2012).

345. Lagiou, P. *et al.* Low carbohydrate-high protein diet and mortality in a cohort of Swedish women. *J. Intern. Med.* **261**, 366–374 (2007).

346. Unwin, D. & Tobin, S. A patient request for some 'deprescribing'. *BMJ* **351**, h4023 (2015).

347. Unwin, D. & Unwin, J. Low carbohydrate diet to achieve weight loss and improve HbA1c in type 2 diabetes and pre-diabetes: experience from one general practice. *Practical Diabetes* https://www.practicaldiabetes.com/article/low-

carbohydrate-diet-achieve-weight-loss-improve-hba1c-type-2-diabetes-pre-diabetes-experience-one-general-practice/.

348.   Fung, T. T. *et al.* Low-carbohydrate diets and all-cause and cause-specific mortality: two cohort studies. *Ann. Intern. Med.* **153**, 289–298 (2010).

349.   Halton, T. L. *et al.* Low-carbohydrate-diet score and the risk of coronary heart disease in women. *N. Engl. J. Med.* **355**, 1991–2002 (2006).

350.   Association between dietary whole grain intake and risk of mortality: two large prospective studies in US men and women. - PubMed - NCBI. https://www.ncbi.nlm.nih.gov/pubmed/25559238.

351.   Li, M. & Shi, Z. A Prospective Association of Nut Consumption with Cognitive Function in Chinese Adults aged 55+ _ China Health and Nutrition Survey. *J Nutr Health Aging* **23**, 211–216 (2019).

352.   Grosso, G. & Estruch, R. Nut consumption and age-related disease. *Maturitas* **84**, 11–16 (2016).

353.   Nugent, S. *et al.* Relationship of metabolic and endocrine parameters to brain glucose metabolism in older adults: do cognitively-normal older adults have a particular metabolic phenotype? *Biogerontology* **17**, 241–255 (2016).

354.   Blueberry-induced changes in spatial working memory correlate with changes in hippocampal CREB phosphorylation and brain-derived neurotrophic facto... - PubMed - NCBI. https://www.ncbi.nlm.nih.gov/pubmed/18457678.

355.   Lautenschlager, N. T. *et al.* Effect of physical activity on cognitive function in older adults at risk for Alzheimer disease: a randomized trial. *JAMA* **300**, 1027–1037 (2008).

356.   Exercise-linked FNDC5/irisin rescues synaptic plasticity and memory defects in Alzheimer's models | Nature Medicine. https://www.nature.com/articles/s41591-018-0275-4.

357.   Tajiri, N. *et al.* Exercise exerts neuroprotective effects on Parkinson's disease model of rats. *Brain research* **1310**, 200–7 (2009).

358.   pubmeddev & al, van N. M., et. Physical inactivity in Parkinson's disease. - PubMed - NCBI. https://sci-hub.tw/https://www.ncbi.nlm.nih.gov/pubmed/?term=216 14433.

359.   Preliminary Report on the Feasibility and Efficacy of the Modified Atkins Diet for Treatment of Mild Cognitive Impairment and Early Alzheimer's Dis... - PubMed - NCBI. https://www.ncbi.nlm.nih.gov/pubmed/30856112.

360.   Phillips, M. C. L., Murtagh, D. K. J., Gilbertson, L. J., Asztely, F. J. S. & Lynch, C. D. P. Low-fat versus ketogenic diet in Parkinson's disease: A pilot randomized controlled trial. *Mov. Disord.* **33**, 1306–1314 (2018).

361.   Krikorian, R. *et al.* Nutritional ketosis for mild cognitive impairment in Parkinson's disease: A controlled pilot trial. *Clinical Parkinsonism & Related Disorders* **1**, 41–47 (2019).

362.   Villemagne, V. L. *et al.* Amyloid β deposition, neurodegeneration, and cognitive decline in sporadic Alzheimer's disease: a prospective cohort study. *Lancet Neurol* **12**, 357–367 (2013).

363.   Shrivastava, A. N. *et al.* Clustering of Tau fibrils impairs the synaptic composition of α3-Na+/K+-ATPase and AMPA receptors. *EMBO J.* **38**, (2019).

364.   Readhead, B. *et al.* Multiscale Analysis of Independent Alzheimer's Cohorts Finds Disruption of

Molecular, Genetic, and Clinical Networks by Human Herpesvirus. *Neuron* **99**, 64-82.e7 (2018).

365.   The Gut and Parkinson's Disease: Hype or Hope? - PubMed   -   NCBI. https://www.ncbi.nlm.nih.gov/pubmed/30584161.

366.   Roth, G. A. *et al.* Global, Regional, and National Burden of Cardiovascular Diseases for 10 Causes, 1990 to 2015. *J. Am. Coll. Cardiol.* **70**, 1–25 (2017).

367.   Epidemiology of Cardiovascular Disease in the 21st Century: Updated Numbers and Updated Facts | Request PDF. https://www.researchgate.net/publication/242487985_Epi demiology_of_Cardiovascular_Disease_in_the_21st_Cent ury_Updated_Numbers_and_Updated_Facts.

368.   Franco, O. H. *et al.* Effects of physical activity on life expectancy with cardiovascular disease. *Arch. Intern. Med.* **165**, 2355–2360 (2005).

369.   Miller, V. *et al.* Estimated Global, Regional, and National Cardiovascular Disease Burdens Related to Fruit and Vegetable Consumption: An Analysis from the Global Dietary Database (FS01-01-19). *Curr Dev Nutr* **3**, (2019).

370.   Millar, C. L., Duclos, Q. & Blesso, C. N. Effects of Dietary Flavonoids on Reverse Cholesterol Transport, HDL Metabolism, and HDL Function. *Adv Nutr* **8**, 226–239 (2017).

371.   Houston, M. C. The importance of potassium in managing hypertension. *Curr. Hypertens. Rep.* **13**, 309–317 (2011).

372.   Whole Fruits and Fruit Fiber Emerging Health Effects.   -   PubMed   -   NCBI. https://www.ncbi.nlm.nih.gov/pubmed/30487459.

373.   Chai, S. C. *et al.* Daily apple versus dried plum: impact on cardiovascular disease risk factors in

postmenopausal women. *J Acad Nutr Diet* **112**, 1158–1168 (2012).
374.	Atorvastatin for lowering lipids. https://www.ncbi.nlm.nih.gov/pmc/articles/PMC6464917/
.
375.	Yamada, T. *et al.* Frequency of citrus fruit intake is associated with the incidence of cardiovascular disease: the Jichi Medical School cohort study. *J Epidemiol* **21**, 169–175 (2011).
376.	Sabaté, J., Oda, K. & Ros, E. Nut consumption and blood lipid levels: a pooled analysis of 25 intervention trials. *Arch. Intern. Med.* **170**, 821–827 (2010).
377.	González, C. A. & Salas-Salvadó, J. The potential of nuts in the prevention of cancer. *Br. J. Nutr.* **96 Suppl 2**, S87-94 (2006).
378.	Kelly, J. H. & Sabaté, J. Nuts and coronary heart disease: an epidemiological perspective. *Br. J. Nutr.* **96 Suppl 2**, S61-67 (2006).
379.	Leung Yinko, S. S. L., Stark, K. D., Thanassoulis, G. & Pilote, L. Fish Consumption and Acute Coronary Syndrome: A Meta-Analysis. *The American Journal of Medicine* **127**, 848-857.e2 (2014).
380.	Fish consumption and risk of stroke and its subtypes: accumulative evidence from a meta-analysis of prospective cohort studies. - PubMed - NCBI. https://www.ncbi.nlm.nih.gov/pubmed/23031847.
381.	Jacques, P. F., Lyass, A., Massaro, J. M., Vasan, R. S. & D'Agostino, R. B. Relationship of lycopene intake and consumption of tomato products to incident CVD. *Br. J. Nutr.* **110**, 545–551 (2013).
382.	Cheng, H. M. *et al.* Lycopene and tomato and risk of cardiovascular diseases: A systematic review and meta-analysis of epidemiological evidence. *Crit Rev Food Sci Nutr* **59**, 141–158 (2019).

383.	Vilahur, G. *et al.* Intake of cooked tomato sauce preserves coronary endothelial function and improves apolipoprotein A-I and apolipoprotein J protein profile in high-density lipoproteins. *Transl Res* **166**, 44–56 (2015).
384.	Block of the Mevalonate Pathway Triggers Oxidative and Inflammatory Molecular Mechanisms Modulated by Exogenous Isoprenoid Compounds. https://www.ncbi.nlm.nih.gov/pmc/articles/PMC4013665/.
385.	Chiva-Blanch, G. & Visioli, F. Polyphenols and health: Moving beyond antioxidants. *Journal of Berry Research* **2**, 63–71 (2012).
386.	He, S.-Y. *et al.* Effect of crocin on experimental atherosclerosis in quails and its mechanisms. *Life Sci.* **77**, 907–921 (2005).
387.	Varshney, R. & Budoff, M. J. Garlic and Heart Disease. *J Nutr* **146**, 416S-421S (2016).
388.	Mellen, P. B., Walsh, T. F. & Herrington, D. M. Whole grain intake and cardiovascular disease: a meta-analysis. *Nutr Metab Cardiovasc Dis* **18**, 283–290 (2008).
389.	Sharma, L., Lou, C., Cahue, S. & Dunlop, D. D. The mechanism of the effect of obesity in knee osteoarthritis: the mediating role of malalignment. *Arthritis Rheum.* **43**, 568–575 (2000).
390.	King, L. K., March, L. & Anandacoomarasamy, A. Obesity & osteoarthritis. *Indian J Med Res* **138**, 185–193 (2013).